Fundamentals of Qualitative Phenomenological Nursing Research

Fundamentals of Qualitative Phenomenological Nursing Research

Brigitte S. Cypress, EdD, RN, CCRN
Rutgers University School of Nursing
Camden, New Jersey, USA

WILEY Blackwell

Registered Offices
John Wiley & Sons, Inc., 111 River Street, Hoboken, NJ 07030, USA
John Wiley & Sons Ltd, The Atrium, Southern Gate, Chichester, West Sussex, PO19 8SQ, UK

Editorial Office
9600 Garsington Road, Oxford, OX4 2DQ, UK

For details of our global editorial offices, customer services, and more information about Wiley products visit us at www.wiley.com.

Wiley also publishes its books in a variety of electronic formats and by print-on-demand. Some content that appears in standard print versions of this book may not be available in other formats.

Limit of Liability/Disclaimer of Warranty
The contents of this work are intended to further general scientific research, understanding, and discussion only and are not intended and should not be relied upon as recommending or promoting scientific method, diagnosis, or treatment by physicians for any particular patient. In view of ongoing research, equipment modifications, changes in governmental regulations, and the constant flow of information relating to the use of medicines, equipment, and devices, the reader is urged to review and evaluate the information provided in the package insert or instructions for each medicine, equipment, or device for, among other things, any changes in the instructions or indication of usage and for added warnings and precautions. While the publisher and authors have used their best efforts in preparing this work, they make no representations or warranties with respect to the accuracy or completeness of the contents of this work and specifically disclaim all warranties, including without limitation any implied warranties of merchantability or fitness for a particular purpose. No warranty may be created or extended by sales representatives, written sales materials or promotional statements for this work. The fact that an organization, website, or product is referred to in this work as a citation and/or potential source of further information does not mean that the publisher and authors endorse the information or services the organization, website, or product may provide or recommendations it may make. This work is sold with the understanding that the publisher is not engaged in rendering professional services. The advice and strategies contained herein may not be suitable for your situation. You should consult with a specialist where appropriate. Further, readers should be aware that websites listed in this work may have changed or disappeared between when this work was written and when it is read. Neither the publisher nor authors shall be liable for any loss of profit or any other commercial damages, including but not limited to special, incidental, consequential, or other damages.

Library of Congress Cataloging-in-Publication Data

Names: Cypress, Brigitte S., author.
Title: Fundamentals of qualitative phenomenological nursing research /
    Brigitte S. Cypress.
Description: Hoboken, NJ : Wiley-Blackwell, 2022. |
    Includes bibliographical references and index.
Identifiers: LCCN 2021032002 (print) | LCCN 2021032003 (ebook) |
    ISBN 9781119780076 (paperback) | ISBN 9781119780083 (Adobe PDF) |
    ISBN 9781119780090 (epub)
Subjects: MESH: Clinical Nursing Research–methods | Nursing Theory |
    Qualitative Research | Research Design
Classification: LCC RT81.5 (print) | LCC RT81.5 (ebook) | NLM WY 20.5 |
    DDC 610.73072–dc23
LC record available at https://lccn.loc.gov/2021032002
LC ebook record available at https://lccn.loc.gov/2021032003

Cover Design: Wiley
Cover Image: © Mina De La O/Getty Images

Set in 10/13pt STIXTwoText by Straive, Pondicherry, India

To my mother, Rosario "Charito" Sia Cypress, who is not with us anymore, "Nay" this is for you. . .

Contents

7 Publishing Qualitative Phenomenological Research Findings ... 114
Kathleen Ahern Gould

About the Author

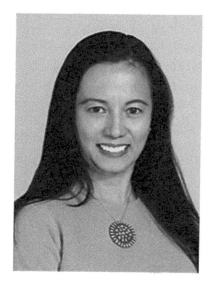

Dr. Brigitte S. Cypress is an Associate Professor at Rutgers, The State University of New Jersey, School of Nursing, Camden. She received her Bachelor of Science nursing degree from Far Eastern University in Manila, Philippines and her Master's degree in Adult Health from Lehman College, City University of New York. Her Doctor of Education degree in nursing is from Teachers College Columbia University, where she began her research program on the lived experience of patients, their family members, and nurses during critical illness.

Using phenomenological philosophy and methods in her research, she continuously conducts studies in critical care that values individuals, specifically the patient-family–nurse relationship, which embraces a holistic approach to the person. Based on the findings of her phenomenological inquiries, she works to develop nursing knowledge essential to the art, philosophy, and practice of the profession, and of healthcare as a whole. She focuses on describing the utility and outcomes of her study findings, and linking them to evidence-based practice, policy, and theory through concept analysis, evidence-based reviews using "meaning questions," and metasynthesis, including generating hypotheses to use in quantitative and mixed-methods research. She believes that phenomenology-as-philosophy and a qualitative research approach are beneficial to qualitative nurse researchers and academicians. Phenomenology can help illuminate and clarify fundamental issues in healthcare through conducting studies into different phenomena evident in nursing practice in the form of lived experiences. As the science of nursing is concerned with treating individuals holistically, phenomenology plays a pivotal role in the profession because it values not only the individual's experience, but also the principles and modalities of their healing into daily life and clinical practice.

The textbook *Fundamentals of Qualitative Phenomenological Nursing Research* by Dr. Brigitte Cypress is a great resource for not only novice researchers, but also anyone who is interested in conducting phenomenological qualitative research. Phenomenological research requires expertise, and this textbook provides a systematic approach from conception to dissemination of a phenomenological qualitative research. Dr. Brigitte Cypress, who has extensive experience in conducting this phenomenological research, has written the textbook in a simple and accessible way.

Dr. Brigitte Cypress' was a professor of mine when I was studying for my PhD in Nursing at the Graduate Center City University of New York. Her passion for philosophy and phenomenological research was evident then, and it shows in her scholarly works. Her vast knowledge and expertise of phenomenological research makes her an authority in this method. Great job Dr. Cypress!

Meriam Caboral-Stevens, PhD, RN, NP-C
Associate Professor
School of Nursing
Eastern Michigan University, Michigan, USA

Dr. Brigitte Cypress is a mentor and educator to PhD students. When I embarked on using phenomenology as the philosophical approach for my dissertation, I called upon her scholarly expertise, and I am honored to have her on my committee. She is an expert when it comes to deciphering and explaining the nuances between all of the different philosophical and phenomenological paradigms, which this textbook so aptly covers.

Dr. Cypress established my foundation as a PhD student and piqued my interest in philosophy and using phenomenology to answer my research question. She was my first professor when I commenced my PhD journey at Pace University. Thank you, Dr Cypress, for all of your patience as I stumble through learning the complicated material, finding my way as a scholar, and for writing this book.

Cindy Paradiso MA, RN-BC, CNE
PhD candidate
Adjunct Clinical Professor
Pace University, New York, USA

With a contribution from

Kathleen Ahern Gould, PhD, MSN, RN
Editor-in-Chief
Dimensions of Critical Care Nursing
Wolters Kluwer/Lippincott
Philadelphia, Pennsylvania, USA

Clinical/Adjunct Faculty
William F. Connell School of Nursing
Boston College
Chestnut Hill, Massachusetts, USA

Foreword

D r. Cypress brings together a seamless pathway to understand the foundation of qualitative research which lays the groundwork for the phenomenological research method. As the utilization of qualitative research approaches continues to expand in nursing and health sciences research, doctoral students and qualitative researchers need to be able to keep abreast of the expanding knowledge, skills, and tools about advances in the foundations of qualitative research and, for many, phenomenological research which supports the development of nursing knowledge. She emphasizes the concepts, methods, instructions/guides, while using an empathetic approach to conduct phenomenological study. The use of real-life exemplars based on self-conducted studies guides the reader through the process of qualitative research with an emphasis on the phenomenological research method. Her approach to phenomenology applies the philosophical aspects in phenomenological studies. This book promotes the understanding and challenges encountered in conducting qualitative and phenomenological approach studies.

As a researcher, professor, and author, Dr. Cypress assists those who are curious about lived experience and links qualitative research to evidence-based practice, policy, theory, and "praxis" (outcomes). Her experience as teacher, researcher, and mentor sheds light on the real challenges in conducting a qualitative study and using data analysis software, all in one book. An exceptional strength of the book is the presentation of exemplars from Dr. Cypress's own research that serve as models for specific phases of phenomenological research process as well as a unique approach to concept analysis, laying a foundation for future research. This book provides the philosophical and paradigmatic aspects of phenomenological research while using exemplars of the application of philosophy to the qualitative research process.

Keville Frederickson, EdD, RN, FAAN
Professor and Founding Director, PhD Program
Lienhard School of Nursing
College of Health Professions
Pace University, New York, USA

Donna M. Nickitas, PhD, RN, NEA-BC, CNE, FNAP, FAAN
Dean and Professor
Rutgers School of Nursing, Camden, New Jersey, USA

List of Tables and Figures

Tables

Figures

Preface

Quoting the title of Wanda Pillow's writing in Merriam's (2002) book, "Looking Back to Move Forward: Reflections on How I Did Research Impacts What I Know Now," this is how I want to start this book: to look back at how I conducted my first qualitative phenomenological research, 11 years ago – my lived experiences of it; the many years of intensive, non-stop reading and learning; meeting with experts; networking with philosophers, phenomenologists, scholars, and researchers of qualitative research; presenting multiple times in conferences around the world; teaching and mentoring undergraduate and graduate students about research; being in dissertation committees of my PhD students; how I grew and flourished in this field and expertise – to become today a phenomenologist, qualitative researcher, scholar, and professor. I have been trained and I prepared well to write this book. Eleven years of phenomenological research: conducting inquiries, writing and applying for grants, writing and publishing consistently through the years – which is not so easy to do, and also not for everyone. The experience has been tedious, intense at times, but rewarding as well, and it becomes part of one's life. Philosophy and phenomenology are what I am passionate about.

As a professor of research at all levels for 13 years now, and as a committee member of qualitative research dissertations, I enjoy guiding and mentoring students in the long and difficult journey of conducting a qualitative inquiry. I am always honest that it is not easy, in fact rather difficult, and could consume one's life. But if it is really what a novice researcher plans for and would love to do, it is also exciting and gratifying. Starting with the hardest step of research, selecting a topic, the question is: "What will I study?" – this could take months or even years to answer, with the new researcher unable to figure out a topic. A lot of times, once a topic is thought of, the novice changes it again and again (which is also normal!). I have a renewed appreciation of the fact that I love to mentor and teach my students that to start delving into a naturalistic study, a "good" mentor is needed. It might not be the chair of the dissertation committee, but the chair can also be one. No doctoral student is fully prepared to go about the methods of a qualitative phenomenological research project, which are: writing the research proposal and getting it approved by the institutional review board (IRB); selecting a setting; obtaining ethical approval; gaining entry to the site; recruiting participants; interviewing and observing participants; writing field notes, journals, and memos; and the hard tasks of data reduction and analysis – not to forget doing the "write-up" later, and trying to publish the findings. All are agonizing tasks! Dissertation templates and protocols are given to students, but these are not sufficient to guide them in this daunting and overwhelming project.

I have seen firsthand the "agony" and difficulty of my doctoral students through the years of being in dissertation committees, and have witnessed the work of novice qualitative researchers. As a reviewer of journals for many years, I have also seen the variations, bewilderment, and confusion with qualitative methodology and methods, especially phenomenology. I continuously see it still. It inspired me to write this book. I intend that the text will be a one-stop resource that can be used by those planning to embark on a qualitative phenomenological study. By all means, this book is not perfect nor an exhaustive reference, but rather a simple, straightforward, and honest guide for new phenomenological researchers and experts alike. Aside from research methods per se, I include topics about the use of data analysis software, phenomenological writing and publishing (including practical tips and recommendations regarding the challenges and dilemmas in conducting phenomenological research), and effective mentoring relationships. What is unique to this book is the articulation and discussion of the outcomes of phenomenological qualitative research: linking findings to evidence-based practice, policy, theory, and theory development, all in one resource that includes actual exemplars.

As I reflect back on how I did my first research, it does impact what I know now. The biggest flaw I continuously see in phenomenological studies is the confusion between phenomenology-as-philosophy (PP) and phenomenology-as-qualitative research (PQR). No one has discussed these two terms more eloquently than John Paley, a colleague at my group – the International Philosophy of Nursing Society (IPONS). He stated these two terms and acronyms in his 2018 book, *Phenomenology as Qualitative Research: A Critical Analysis of Meaning Attribution*, as he rigorously analyzed the methodological aspect of research studies in the literature using the approaches of experts and PQR methodologists like Amedeo Giorgi, Max van Manen, Jonathan Smith, Paul Flowers, and Michael Larkin. A lot of phenomenological inquiries I have read in the literature are labeled as "phenomenological" but on closer attention to the methods prove to be short of what a correct phenomenological study should be. When I say "methods," I am referring to the philosophical stance, paradigmatic underpinnings, and approach that are evident in the application of methods of data collection, phenomenological reduction, analysis, and rigor. The debate about PP versus PQR continues to this day. More so, the criticisms by other disciplines of the nursing discipline's "faulty" use of phenomenology as a research method seem to be never-ending and are still evident.

I cannot forget the first time I presented the findings of my first phenomenological study 10 years ago, to an audience of phenomenologists, philosophers, and scholars of qualitative research from different countries. Not that I was nervous – but I was anticipating what these experts would ask me about the study (mostly on phenomenology) and how I conducted the research. The president of the group (whom I had great respect for, and who is now deceased) stated, "Okay kiddo, let's hear it!" – and he sat in the front row. After my presentation, I was amazed that he actually said to the audience that he appreciated very much having me as the only nurse member in the group, and that he wished that more nurses would try to present in the conference in the future, or become a member of the organization. He did not ask me questions (maybe because it was my first time and he decided to cut me some slack!). In the many years that I presented in conferences after that first one, I was gradually asked respectfully the questions specific to phenomenology as a qualitative research method in nursing studies. I tried answering based on what I knew and had experienced. My answers got better after many years of learning. This is one of the ways in which I learned the right way of conducting a phenomenological study: answering the questions and applying them to my work. Other issues I have been asked about are specific to the methods.

The other big aspects of phenomenological research that are many times put into question are the never-ending issues with rigor and the techniques of sampling, bracketing, and data saturation. My work on these aspects continues. All these steps/techniques, the biggest question on phenomenology-as-research, and how to conduct the research correctly – I cannot blame students and novices for stumbling at these hurdles. They are the hardest topics for me to write about in this book. One significant contributing factor is the lack of knowledge of philosophy, because philosophy is not taught, or is not included in the undergraduate and graduate (master's level) curriculum, at most nursing schools. Even at the doctorate level, there is only one philosophy course – which is labeled differently in every school (philosophy of science, philosophies of education, philosophical and theory perspectives in nursing, and many others), and taught in varied ways. One philosophy course at the doctorate level is not sufficient to equip a neophyte researcher for a qualitative phenomenological study. I only learned all the details after being exposed to my philosophy colleagues, co-phenomenologists, and other scholars from different parts of the world. Eleven years of networking, countless discussions and consultations, presenting in conferences, being critiqued and learning from and with colleagues in seminars, including endless and continuous reading of philosophical texts – all that to reach what I know now. I am still continuously learning, and I don't intend to stop.

Philosophy and phenomenology are difficult for students and novices embarking for the first time on a journey of phenomenological study. There is no chance, I would say, that philosophy will be taught more in curriculums in the future (although there are a few schools with curriculums that are more focused on philosophy, and even phenomenology). Thus, a novice or graduate student has to be interested, motivated, and passionate, learn on their own, read a whole lot, try to understand and apply the knowledge gained to the endeavor – but guidance is needed. This is where a "good" mentor comes in. I would hope that the mentor first has a background in conducting qualitative studies as a whole, and more importantly, has some knowledge of philosophy and phenomenology. As we all know, there are very few professors in nursing who like and teach philosophy, which sometimes results in the course being taught by faculty from the philosophy department. Philosophy professors, of course, are experts in philosophy per se – but there is a bit of a disconnect sometimes in how to link philosophy to nursing. I taught and co-taught philosophy in the doctorate level with amazing colleagues from both philosophy and nursing for many years. I still have some questions about how philosophy per se and philosophy-as-research should be presented to students who will be embarking on the difficult journey of phenomenological study. This became my inspiration for writing the chapters on philosophical and paradigmatic aspects, rigor, and challenges and dilemmas, including effective mentoring relationships. I remind my students that as they continue on their odyssey, they will make mistakes – but with the help of a qualified, respectful, understanding, flexible, and patient mentor, they will get through them and complete the research project. It will not be a "smooth ride" – but one with unpredictable "ebbs and flows." Wanda is right, "looking back and reflecting on how I did research impacts what I know now, and how I will move forward."

Brigitte S. Cypress
Rutgers University School of Nursing
Camden, New Jersey, USA

Acknowledgments

I would like to sincerely thank Wiley for publishing this book.

I gratefully acknowledge permission from Sage, Taylor and Francis, Springer, BMJ Publishing Group, and Wiley for the following sources:

Alexander, R.K., Diefenbeck, C.A., and Brown, C.B. (2015). Career choice and longevity in U.S. psychiatric–mental health nurses. *Issues in Mental Health Nursing* 36 (6): 447–454.

Creswell, J.W. and Poth, C.N. (2017). *Qualitative Inquiry & Research Design: Choosing Among Five Approaches*, 4e. Sage Publications.

Elliott, R.A, Lee, C.Y., Beanland, C. et al. (2017). Development of a clinical pharmacy model within an Australian home nursing service using co-creation and participatory action research: the *Visiting Pharmacist* (ViP) study. *BMJ Open* 7: e018722, 1–10.

Giorgi, A. (2008). Concerning a serious misunderstanding of the essence of the phenomenological method in psychology. *Journal of Phenomenological Psychology* 39: 33–58.

Patton, M.Q. (2014). *Qualitative Research and Methods: Integrating Theory and Practice*, 4e. Sage Publications.

Silverman, D. (2005). *Doing Qualitative Research*, 2e. Sage Publications.

St. John, W. and Johnson, P. (2000). The pros and cons of data analysis software for qualitative research. *Journal of Nursing Scholarship* 32 (4): 393–394.

Tolman, D., Hirschman, C., and Impett, E.A. (2005). There is more to the story: the place of qualitative research on female adolescent sexuality in policy making. *Sexuality Research and Social Policy: Journal of NSRC* 2 (4): 4–17.

Whittemore, R., Chase, S.K., and Mandle, C.L. (2001). Validity in qualitative research. *Qualitative Health Research* 11 (2): 117–132.

Thank you to Dr. Max van Manen for the great ideas in his two books:

Van Manen, M. (2014). *Phenomenology of Practice: Meaning-Giving Methods in Phenomenological Research and Writing*. Left Coast Press.

Van Manen, M. (1990). *Researching Lived Experience: Human Science for an Action Sensitive Pedagogy*. State University Press.

I am grateful to Dr. Janice Morse for her qualitative books:

Morse, J. (2012). *Qualitative Health Research: Creating a New Discipline*. Left Coast Press.

Morse, J. (2012). *Qualitative Health Research: Creating a New Discipline*, 1e. Routledge.

Morse, J., Swanson, J.J., and Kuzel, A.J. (2001). *The Nature of Qualitative Evidence*. Sage Publications.

Morse, J. (1997). *Completing a Qualitative Project: Details and Dialogue*. Sage Publications.

Morse, J. and Field, P.A. (1995). *Qualitative Research Methods for Health Professionals*, 2e. Sage Publications.

Morse, J. (1994). *Critical Issues in Qualitative Research Methods*. Sage Publications.

Morse, J. (1991). *Qualitative Nursing Research: A Contemporary Dialogue*. Sage Publications.

My sincere gratitude to Dr. Kathleen Ahern Gould for her ideas and suggestions on topics to write and present to our journal audience. The qualitative research methodological article series I wrote for *DCCN* inspired me to write this book. Thank you also for writing Chapter 7 on Publishing Qualitative Phenomenological Research Findings. I am thankful to Dr. Vickie Miracle. I published my first article in that same journal when she was the chief editor. I learned a lot, and honed my writing skills through the years working with both of them. Coincidentally, Wiley (which publishes *DCCN*) accepted my book proposal when I submitted it. I think this is meant to be – that I continue to be working with this great group of experts, and this publishing company.

My heartfelt thanks to Dr. Keville Frederickson and Dr. Donna Nickitas for their mentorship, guidance, support, and friendship through the years. You have always been there for me.

Thank you to Dr. Meriam Caboral-Stevens for the views and thoughts we share, and for your friendship.

The ideas for this text I have pondered, presented, and discussed with colleagues and friends from the International Coalition of North American Phenomenologists (ICNAP), the International Philosophy of Nursing Society (IPONS), and the International Human Science Research Conference (IHSRC) group over the years. I am indebted to all of you who listened, questioned, argued, and gave suggestions for my work. I learned a lot from you all.

To all my research students, for whom I have learned so much – my reason for writing this book is *YOU!*

How to Use this Book

What is this textbook designed to do? As a whole, there are very few phenomenological nursing research textbooks published that are singly authored and offer a one-stop holistic resource for novice researchers, graduate students, and experts alike. This text aims not only to guide qualitative phenomenological researchers on the selection of appropriate methods and techniques (as many books in the literature already do) but also to provide detailed discussions about rigor and the philosophical, paradigmatic, and conceptual aspects of phenomenological research, with full exemplars in each case drawn from my own studies. It also includes practical tips on the use of data analysis software, writing, publishing, the importance of mentoring relationships, and the challenges and dilemmas facing new researchers when they conduct a phenomenological inquiry. This will be the first qualitative book that presents the outcomes of qualitative research and specifically links them to evidence-based practice, policy, theory, and theory development – all in one resource.

I started by sharing in the Preface my *lived* experience of conducting my first phenomenological study, looking back to how I continuously learned and grew through the years using this qualitative research methodology, how it impacted what I know now, and how I applied the knowledge I gained moving forward.

This book is divided into six parts. Part I first describes qualitative research as a whole, and then more specifically examines the philosophical, paradigmatic, and conceptual underpinnings of phenomenological inquiry. Part II looks at the methods of phenomenological data collection, reduction, analysis, interpretation, and presentation. Part III focuses on enhancing rigor and validity in phenomenological studies. Part IV provides a description of phenomenological writing, reporting, and publishing. Part V is about the practical aspects of phenomenological investigations. Finally, Part VI deals with phenomenological outcomes and applications in evidence-based practice, policy, theory, and theory development.

Chapter 1 presents a snapshot of what qualitative research is and what its components are, before delving into the specifics of phenomenological philosophy and methodology.

Chapter 2 discusses methods appropriate for conducting a qualitative phenomenological research study that evolves from philosophical, paradigmatic, inductive, and conceptual perspectives. It includes a discussion of the philosophers Edmund Husserl, Martin Heidegger, and Maurice Merleau-Ponty, and offers phenomenological studies applying the methods of Merleau-Ponty, Giorgi, and van Manen as exemplars.

Chapter 3 discusses ethical issues, means and methods for collecting, recording, and securely storing data, approaches to data analysis, the organization, reading, and coding of themes, and the representation and interpretation of data. It looks at potential unanticipated issues in each of these areas, and offers appropriate solutions.

Chapter 4 examines the role of computer-assisted qualitative data analysis software, focusing on the methodological issues surrounding program use. It offers a brief review of two very common and widely used qualitative data analysis software packages.

Chapter 5 deals with the concept of rigor in qualitative research, using a phenomenological study as an exemplar. Elaborating on epistemological and theoretical conceptualizations, it makes recommendations for the renewed use of the concepts of reliability and validity in qualitative research.

Chapter 6 looks at the importance of writing in phenomenological research, including ethical considerations, approaches, techniques, and structures.

Chapter 7 describes approaches to publishing qualitative phenomenological findings, including finding the right journal, understanding publishing contracts, working with editors, navigating the peer-review and production processes, writing and revising manuscripts, understanding modes of publishing, and marketing one's work.

Chapter 8 illuminates the challenges and dilemmas of a phenomenological inquiry. It makes recommendations and offers approaches in order to better address these issues.

Chapter 9 introduces the role of mentoring in successfully completing a phenomenological research project, in order to help equip novices with the requisite knowledge, skills, and confidence and thus empower them to navigate the difficult and long journey of a qualitative investigation.

Chapter 10 describes the utility of qualitative research findings and their linkage to outcomes – specifically, to evidence-based practice (EBP), policy, theory, and theory development. It presents two exemplar evidence-based reviews using "meaning questions," and addresses approaches to policy, theory, and theory development using exemplars from research investigations and my own metasynthesis study of family presence.

Ultimately, no book is perfect, but as an author, researcher, and phenomenologist, I aim that the text will afford some clarity and help to all investigators of qualitative phenomenological inquiry.

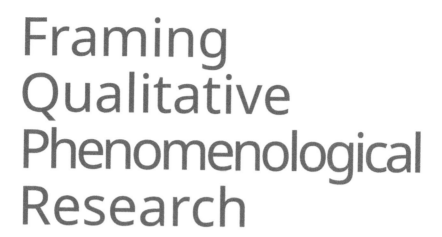

Framing Qualitative Phenomenological Research

1

The "What," "Why," "Who," and "How" of Qualitative Research
A Snapshot

Qualitative research methods began to appear in nursing in the 1960s and 1970s, to cautious and reluctant acceptance. In the 1980s, qualitative health research emerged as a distinctive domain and mode of inquiry (Sandelowski 2003). "Qualitative research" refers to any kind of research that produces findings not arrived at by means of statistical analysis or other means of quantification (Borbasi and Jackson 2012; Strauss and Corbin 1990). It uses a naturalistic approach that seeks to understand phenomena related to persons' lives, stories, and behaviors, including those related to health, organizational functioning, social movements, and interactional relationships. It is underpinned by several theoretical perspectives, namely constructivist-interpretive, critical, post-positivist, post-structural/post-modern, and feminist (Ingham-Broomfield 2015). One conducts a qualitative study to uncover the nature of a person's experiences with a phenomenon in context-specific conditions such as illness (acute and chronic), addiction, loss, disability, and end-of-life (**EOL**). Qualitative research is used to explore, uncover, describe, and understand what lies behind a given phenomenon, about which little may be known. This deeper understanding can only be attained through a qualitative inquiry, and not through mere numbers or statistical models. Qualitative inquiry represents a legitimate mode of social and human science exploration, without apology and without comparison to quantitative research (Creswell 2007).

1.1 Why Do Qualitative Research?

The tradition of using qualitative methods to study human phenomena is grounded in the social sciences (Streubert and Carpenter 1999). This methodological revolution has made way for a more interpretative approach, because aspects of human values, culture, and relationships are not described fully using quantitative research methods. Unlike quantitative researchers, who seek causal determination, prediction, and generalization of findings, qualitative researchers allow the phenomenon of interest to unfold naturally (Patton 2014), striving to explore, describe, understand, and delve into a colorful, deep, contextual world of interpretations (Golafshani 2001). Thus, the practice of qualitative research has expanded to clinical settings because empirical approaches have proven to be inadequate in answering questions related to human subjectivity where interpretation is

Fundamentals of Qualitative Phenomenological Nursing Research, First Edition. Brigitte S. Cypress.
© 2022 John Wiley & Sons Ltd. Published 2022 by John Wiley & Sons Ltd.

involved (Thorne 1997). Consequently, qualitative health research is a research approach to exploring health and illness as they are perceived by the individual, rather than from the researcher's perspective (Morse 2012). Morse (2012) states that "Researchers use qualitative research methods to illicit emotions and perspectives, beliefs, and values, actions, and behaviors, and to understand the participant's responses to health and illness, and the meanings they construct about the experience" (p. 21). Qualitative research provides a rich inductive description that necessitates interpretation. It also calls for more holistic evidence to inform health policy decision-making, shining a spotlight on the synthesis of qualitative evidence (Carroll 2017; Lewin et al. 2018; Majid and Vanstone 2018). Researchers in the healthcare arena, practitioners, and policy-makers are increasingly pressed to translate these qualitative findings for practice, put them to use, and evaluate their utility in effecting desired change, with the goal of improving public health and reducing disparities in healthcare delivery (Sandelowski 2003).

Morse (2012) asserts that there are other reasons for conducting a qualitative inquiry. Other writers believe that the role of qualitative inquiry is to provide hypotheses and research questions based on the findings of qualitative studies. Qualitative research can serve as a foundation from which to develop surveys and questionnaires, thus producing models for quantitative testing. But what is really the most important function of qualitative inquiry? According to Morse (2012), it is the moral imperative of qualitative inquiry to *humanize* health care. She states: "The social justice agenda of qualitative health research is one that *humanizes* health care" (p. 52). So, what is *humanizing* health care? Morse (2012) articulates: "Humanizing encompasses a perspective on attitudes, beliefs, expectations, practices, and behaviors that influence the quality of care, administration of that care, conditions judged to warrant (or not warrant) empathetic care, responses to care, and therapeutics, and anticipated and actual outcomes of patient or community care" (pp. 54–55).

Conducting research should be sort of a social justice project. Denzin (2010) recognizes making social justice a public agenda within qualitative inquiry. He emphasizes that qualitative inquiry can contribute to social justice through: (i) identifying different definitions of a problem and/or situation that is being evaluated with some agreement that change is required; (ii) locating the assumptions held by policy-makers, clients, welfare workers, online professionals, and other interested parties and showing them to be correct or incorrect; (iii) identifying the strategic points of interventions and thus enabling them to be evaluated and improved; (iv) suggesting alternative moral points of view from which the problem, the policy, and the program can be interpreted and assessed; and (v) exposing the limits of statistics and statistical evaluations using the more qualitative materials furnished by this approach (pp. 24–25).

1.2 Who Does Qualitative Research?

Qualitative research is done by researchers in the social sciences, as well as by practitioners in fields that concern themselves with issues related to human behavior and functioning. These are health professionals who are able to identify a research question and recognize the particular context and situation that will achieve the best answers to it. According to Morse (2012), the qualitative health researcher should be an expert methodologist who has an understanding of illness, the patient's condition, and staff roles and relationships, and who can balance the clinical situation from different perspectives (p. 23). A qualitative researcher also requires theoretical and social sensibility, interactional skills, the ability to maintain analytical distance while drawing upon past experience, and theoretical knowledge to interpret what they observe.

1.3 What Are the Characteristics of Qualitative Research?

Creswell (2012) discusses how qualitative research studies today involve closer attention to the interpretive nature of inquiry, and situation within the political, social, and cultural context of the researchers, participants, and readers. He presents several characteristics of qualitative research, as follows: (i) natural setting: data are collected face-to-face in the field at the site where participants experience the phenomenon under study; the inquiry should also be conducted in a way that does not disturb the natural context of the phenomenon; (ii) researcher as key instrument: the researchers collect the data themselves rather than relying on instruments developed by others; (iii) multiple sources of data: the researchers gather multiple forms of data, including interviews, observations, and document examination, rather than rely on a single source; (iv) inductive data analysis: data are organized into abstract units of information ("bottom-up" or moving from specific to general), working back and forth between the themes and the database until a comprehensive set of themes is established, and ending up with general conclusions or theories; (v) participant's meanings: the researchers keep a focus on learning the meaning that the participants hold about the phenomenon, and not the meaning that they bring to the study themselves; (vi) emergent design: the initial plan for the study cannot be tightly prescribed, but must be emergent; all phases of the process may change or shift after the researchers enter the field and begin to collect data; (vii) theoretical lens: use of a "lens" to view the study, such as the concept of culture, gender, race, or class differences, or the social, political, or historical context of the problem under study; (viii) interpretive inquiry: a form of inquiry in which the researchers make an interpretation of what they see, hear, and understand, which cannot be separated from their own background, history, context, and prior understanding; and (ix) holistic account: reporting multiple perspectives, identifying the many factors involved in the situation, and sketching the larger picture that emerges (Creswell 2012).

1.4 What Are the Methods Frequently Used in Qualitative Research?

The research question dictates the method to be used for a qualitative study. Qualitative and quantitative questions are distinct, and serve different purposes. Some of the different types of qualitative research that will be discussed in this chapter are: phenomenology, grounded theory, ethnography, case study, and narrative research. Researchers from different disciplines use different approaches depending on what the purpose of their study is.

Narrative research begins with the experiences as expressed in the lived and told stories of individuals. Narrative is a spoken word or written text giving an account of an event/action chronologically connected. Examples of this approach are biographical studies, autobiographies, and life stories. Kvangarsnes et al. (2013) explored patient perceptions of chronic obstructive pulmonary disease (**COPD**) exacerbation and patient experiences of relations with health personnel during care and treatment using narrative research design. They conducted ten in-depth qualitative interviews with patients who had been admitted to two intensive care units (**ICUs**) in Western Norway during the autumn of 2009 and the spring of 2010, and used narrative analysis and theories on trust and power to analyze the results. The patients perceived that they were completely dependent on others during the acute phase. Some stated that they had experienced an altered perception of reality and had not understood how serious their situation was. Although the patients trusted the health personnel in helping them breathe, they also told stories about care deficiencies and situations in which they felt neglected. This study shows that patients with an acute exacerbation of COPD often feel wholly dependent on health personnel during the exacerbation and, as a result, experience extreme vulnerability.

Where a narrative approach explores the life of a single person, a phenomenological study describes the meaning for several individuals of their lived experiences of a phenomenon. Phenomenology is the most inductive of all qualitative methods. It involves the study of the lived experiences of persons, the view that these experiences are conscious ones, and the development of descriptions of the essences of these experiences, not explanations or analysis. There are several different types of phenomenological approach, namely: descriptive-transcendental (Husserl, Giorgi), interpretive/hermeneutic (Heidegger, Gadamer, Jean-Luc Nancy, Van Manen), descriptive-hermeneutic (Merleau-Ponty, van Manen), empirical-transcendental (Moustakas), and existential-embodied (Sarte, Heidegger, Merleau-Ponty). A phenomenological study conducted by Cypress (2014) explored the lived experiences of nurses, patients, and family members during critical illness in an emergency department (**ED**). Data were collected over a six-month period by means of in-depth interviews, and thematic analysis was done using van Manen's (1990) descriptive- hermeneutic phenomenological approach. The findings indicate that the patients' and their family members' perceptions of the nurses in the ED related to their critical thinking skills, communication, sensitivity, and caring abilities. Nurses identified that response to a patient's physiological deficit is paramount in the ED, and that involving the patient and their family in the human care processes will help attain this goal.

While phenomenology aims to illuminate themes and describe the meaning of the lived experiences of a number of individuals, grounded theory attempts to move beyond description and to generate or discover a theory, an abstract analytical schema of a process or interaction shaped by the views of a large number of participants. This qualitative method was developed by Glaser and Strauss in 1967. Other grounded theorists followed, including Clarke (2005), who relies on post-modern perspectives, and Charmaz (2006), who relies on constructivist approach. Gallagher et al. (2015) collected and analyzed qualitative data using grounded theory to understand nurses' EOL decision-making practices in five ICUs in different cultural contexts. Interviews were conducted with 51 experienced ICU nurses on university or hospital premises in five countries. The comparative analysis within and across data generated by the different research teams enabled the researchers to develop a deeper understanding of EOL decision-making practices in the ICU. The core category that emerged was "negotiated reorienting." Gallagher et al. (2015) stated: "Whilst nurses do not make the 'ultimate' EOL decisions, they engage in two core practices: consensus seeking (involving coaxing, information cuing and voice enabling); and emotional holding (creating time-space, and comfort giving)" (p. 794).

Although a grounded theory approach examines a number of individuals to develop a hypothesis, participants are not studied as one unit. Ethnography, meanwhile, uses a larger number of individuals and focuses on an entire cultural group as a single unit of analysis, describing and interpreting their shared and learned patterns of values, behaviors, beliefs, and language. There are many forms of ethnography, namely: confessional, life history, auto-ethnography, feminist, ethnographic novels, visual ethnography found in photography, and video and electronic media. Price (2013) explored what aspects affect registered healthcare professionals' ability to care for patients within the technological environment of a critical care unit. They utilized ethnography to focus on the cultural elements within a given situation. Data collection involved participant observation, document review, and semi-structured interviews with the nineteen study participants. An overarching theme of the "crafting process" was developed, with sub-themes of "vigilance," "focus of attention," "being present," and "expectations," with an ultimate goal of achieving the best interests for the individual patient.

A culture-sharing group in ethnography can be considered a *case*, but its aim is to ascertain how the culture works rather than to understand one or more specific cases within a bounded system. Creswell (2012) defines case study research as an approach in which the researcher explores a bounded system (a case) or multiple bounded systems (cases) over time through detailed in-depth data collection involving multiple sources of information and reports a case description and case-based themes (p. 73). In terms of intent, there are three types of case study: single instrumental, collective or multiple, and intrinsic. Hyde-Wyatt (2014) studied spinally injured patients on sedation in the ICU. A reflection-on-action exercise was carried out when a spinally injured patient became physically active during a sedation hold. This was attributed to hyperactive delirium. Reflection on this incident led to a literature search for guidance on the likelihood of delirium causing secondary spinal injury in patients with unstable fractures. Through a case study approach, the research was reviewed in relation to a particular patient. This case study illustrated that there was a knowledge deficit when it came to managing the combination of the patient's spinal injury and delirium. Sedation cessation episodes are an essential part of patient care in the ICU. For spinally injured patients, these may need to be modified to sedation reductions to prevent sudden wakening and uncontrolled movement should they be experiencing hyperactive delirium.

1.5 What Is the Process of Conceptualizing and Designing a Qualitative Research Inquiry?

Designing a qualitative inquiry is not a fully structured, rigid process. Even books and experts vary in their understanding and guidance. Conducting a qualitative study is extremely difficult (Morse 2012, p. 76). Sometimes, there is concern about access and the qualitative procedures involved in data collection, including disclosure of participants' identities and confidentiality of data. Nevertheless, qualitative research involves a rigorous and scientific process that serves as a guide for researchers who are planning to embark on a journey and complete a naturalistic investigation.

Unlike quantitative research, which involves a fairly linear process, qualitative studies have a flexible approach and flow of activities. The researchers do not know in advance exactly how the study will unfold (Hyde-Wyatt 2014). The process of designing a qualitative study thus does not begin with the methods – which in fact is the easiest part of naturalistic inquiries (Creswell 2012). Qualitative researchers instead usually begin with a broad topic focusing on one aspect of a phenomenon about which little is known. The phenomenon may be one in the "real world," a gap in the literature, or past findings of investigations (e.g., in the area of social and human sciences) (Creswell 2012). A fairly broad question is then posed, in order to allow the focus to be delineated; this can then be sharpened when the study is underway.

Once the research question has been posed, the researchers should conduct a brief literature review to inform the question and to help establish the significance of the problem. There is a continuous debate about the value of doing a literature review prior to collecting data, and how much of one should be done. Some believe that knowledge about findings of previous studies might influence the conceptualization of the phenomenon of interest, which ideally should be illuminated by the participants rather than by prior findings (Polit and Beck 2014). A grounded theory investigator, for example, may make a point of not conducting a review of literature before beginning their study to avoid "contamination" of the data with preconceived concepts and notions about what might be relevant (Borbasi and Jackson 2012).

After the literature review, the researchers must identify an appropriate site for the study. Selecting and gaining entry to a site requires knowledge of settings in which participants in their lifeworld are experiencing the phenomenon under study. For example, research in the area of health is a very broad topic. A researcher should determine definitions, concepts, scopes, and theories about health that will be used for the proposed qualitative inquiry. Health can be perceived as the absence or presence of illness, or as the physical, psychosocial, psychological, or spiritual health of individuals, families, or groups (Morse 2012). Morse (2012) states that "Research into the intimate, experiential and interpersonal aspects of illness, into caring for the ill, and into seeking and maintaining wellness introduces extraordinary methodological challenges" (p. 89). Thus, knowledge about the characteristics of the participants who will be recruited for the study and the specific context of the settings (i.e., hospital/institution, community/outpatient) in which they are located at the time when research will be conducted is important. In order to gain entry to the site, the ethical aspect of the study should also be addressed. Approval from the appropriate institutional review board (**IRB**) and informed consent from the participants must be obtained. Qualitative studies have special ethical concerns because of the more intimate nature of the relationship that typically develop between researchers and participants (Polit and Beck 2014). The researchers must develop specific plans addressing these issues.

After addressing the ethical concerns and gaining entry to the site, an overall approach should be planned and developed. Although the researchers might plan for a specific approach to be used, the design can be emergent during the course of data collection. Modifications may be made as the need arises. It is rare that a qualitative study has a rigidly structured design that prohibits changes while in the field (Polit and Beck 2014), but the purposes, questions, and methods of research must nonetheless be interconnected and interrelated so that the study appears as a cohesive whole rather than fragmented isolated parts (Creswell 2007, p. 42). For example, patients in hospitals have limited abilities related to their medical condition and the contextual features of the hospital setting. A patient's condition may thus demand a different method be used because of fatigue, interruptions due to treatments or physicians' rounds, and visitors. In this context, the study will require modifications of methods, and study participation will have the lowest priority at the specific moment and time (Morse 2012).

In qualitative studies, sampling, data collection, and analysis – including interpretation – take place repetitively. The sampling method usually used is purposive. Qualitative researchers employ rigorous data collection procedures involving interviewing and observing them (individuals, focus groups, or an entire culture) in order to explore the phenomenon under study. The discussions and observations are loosely structured, allowing the participants a full range of beliefs, feelings, and behaviors (Polit and Beck 2014). Other types of information that can be collected are documents, photographs, audio-visual materials, sounds, emails, text messages, and computer software.

The backbone of qualitative research is extensive collection of data from multiple sources (Creswell 2012). After organizing and storing the data, the researchers will try to make sense of them, working inductively from particulars to more general perspectives until categories, codes, and themes emerge and are illuminated, which can be used to build a rich description of the phenomenon of interest (Creswell 2012; Polit and Beck 2014). The researchers will analyze the data using multiple levels of abstraction. Analysis and interpretation are ongoing concurrent activities that guide the researchers on the kinds of questions to ask and the kinds of observations to make. The types of data gathered become increasingly meaningful as the theory emerges. Data collection ceases when the complexity and scope of the phenomenon have been fully explored and varied strategies have been applied according to the nature of the participants and the researchers' expertise with thinking qualitatively (Morse 2020).

Rigor and the trustworthiness of the data have then to be established. Steps must be taken to confirm that the findings accurately reflect the experiences and perceptions of the participants, rather than the viewpoints of the researchers. Some of the strategies that can be used are validation techniques including confirming and triangulating data from several sources, going back to the participants, sharing preliminary interpretations with the participants, asking the participants whether the researchers' thematic analysis is consistent with their experiences (Polit and Beck 2014, p. 55), and having other expert researchers review the procedures undertaken and interpretations made (Creswell 2012).

1.6 Conclusion

Qualitative research uses a naturalistic approach that seeks to understand phenomena in context-specific settings in order to make sense of them and interpret them in terms of the meaning people bring to them. It contributes to the humanizing of healthcare as it addresses topics of health and illness. It does not have firm or rigid guidelines, and it takes time to conduct. Some of the methods that can be used for a qualitative inquiry are narrative research, phenomenology, grounded theory, case study, and ethnography. Although the study design emerges during the inquiry, it follows the pattern of scientific research. Researchers collect data rigorously in natural settings over a period of time and analyze them inductively to establish patterns or themes. Ethical decisions and considerations around rigor and trustworthiness are continuously threaded throughout the study. The final report presents the active voices of participants and a description and interpretation of the meaning of the phenomenon, including the reflexivity of the researcher.

References

Borbasi, S. and Jackson, D. (2012). *Navigating the Maze of Research*. Mosby Elsevier.

Carroll, C. (2017). Qualitative evidence synthesis to improve implementation of clinical guidelines. *British Medical Journal* 356 (j80): 1–4.

Charmaz, K. (2006). *Constructing Grounded Theory: A Practical Guide through Qualitative Analysis*. Sage Publications.

Clarke, A. (2005). *Situational Analysis: Grounded Theory after the Postmodern Turn*. Sage Publications.

Creswell, J.W. (2007). *Qualitative Inquiry and Research Design: Choosing Among Five Approaches*, 2e. Sage Publications.

Creswell, J.W. (2012). *Qualitative Inquiry and Research Design: Choosing Among Five Approaches*, 3e. Sage Publications.

Cypress, B. (2014). The emergency room: experiences of patients, families, and their nurses. *Advanced Emergency Nursing Journal* 36 (2): 164–176.

Denzin, N. (2010). *The Qualitative Manifesto: A Call to Arms*. Left Coast Press.

Glaser, B.G. and Strauss, A.L. (1967). *The Discovery of Grounded Theory: Strategies for Qualitative Research*. Aldine.

Golafshani, N. (2001). Understanding reliability and validity in qualitative research. *The Qualitative Report* 8 (4): 597–607.

Hyde-Wyatt, J.P. (2014). Managing hyperactive delirium and spinal immobilization in the intensive care setting: a case study and reflective discussion of the literature. *Intensive and Critical Care Nursing* 30 (3): 138–144.

Ingham-Broomfield, R. (2015). A nurses' guide to qualitative research. *Australian Journal of Advanced Nursing* 32 (3): 34–40.

International Nurses' End-of-Life Decision-Making in Intensive Care Research Group, Gallagher, A., Bousso, R.S. et al. (2015). Negotiated reorienting: a grounded theory of nurses' end-of-life decision-making in the intensive care unit. *International Journal of Nursing Studies* 52 (4): 794–803.

Kvangarsnes, M., Torheim, H., Hole, T., and Ohlund, L. (2013). Narratives of breathlessness in chronic obstructive pulmonary disease. *Journal of Clinical Nursing* 22 (21–22): 3062–3070.

Lewin, S., Booth, A., Glenton, C. et al. (2018). Applying GRADE-CERQual to qualitative evidence synthesis findings: introduction to the series. *Implementation Science* 13 (2): 1–10.

Majid, U. and Vanstone, M. (2018). Appraising qualitative research for evidence syntheses: a compendium of quality appraisal tools. *Qualitative Health Research* 28 (13): 2115–2131.

Morse, J. (2012). *Qualitative Health Research: Creating a New Discipline*. Left Coast Press.

Morse, J. (2020). The changing face of qualitative inquiry. *International Journal of Qualitative Methods* 19: 1–7.

Patton, M.Q. (2014). *Qualitative Research and Evaluation Methods: Integrating Theory and Practice*, 4e. Sage Publications.

Polit, D.F. and Beck, C.T. (2014). *Essentials of Nursing Research: Appraising Evidence for Nursing Practice*. Wolters Kluwer/Lippincott Williams & Wilkins.

Price, A.M. (2013). Caring and technology in an intensive care unit: an ethnographic study. *British Association of Critical Care Nurses* 18 (6): 278–288.

Sandelowski, M. (2003). Using qualitative research. *Qualitative Health Research* 14 (10): 1386.

Strauss, A. and Corbin, J. (1990). *Basics of Qualitative Research: Grounded Theory Procedures and Techniques*. Sage Publications.

Streubert, H.J. and Carpenter, D.R. (1999). *Qualitative Research in Nursing: Advancing the Humanistic Imperative*, 3e. Lippincott Williams & Wilkins.

Thorne, S. (1997). *The art (and science) of critiquing qualitative research*. In: *Completing a Qualitative Project: Details and Dialogue* (ed. J.M. Morse), 117–132. Sage Publications.

van Manen, M. (1990). *Researching Lived Experience: Human Science for an Action Sensitive Pedagogy*. State University Press.

2 Exploring the Philosophical, Paradigmatic, and Conceptual Underpinnings of Qualitative Phenomenological Research

Qualitative research has made a strong impression on nursing science since the 1990s. This burgeoning interest is not without confusion, controversy, and a lack of consistency of protocols and structure, however (Morse 1991). There is still some work to be done on the refinement and establishment of consistent research methods and guidelines. The key to understanding qualitative research lies with the idea that meaning is socially constructed by individuals in interaction with their world. Qualitative research offers the opportunity to focus on finding answers to questions centered on social experience – how it is created, and how it gives meaning to human life (Streubert and Carpenter 1999). The world or reality is dynamic, and not a fixed, single, or measurable phenomenon. There are multiple constructions, interpretations, and contexts of reality, and it changes over time (Merriam 2002). Recognizing this is the first step in establishing a truly humanistic perspective of qualitative research.

There are issues that arise from the application of qualitative methods for examining nursing phenomena (Morse 1991; Morse et al. 2001). The first question is: Should the research methods used in other disciplines, including assumptions, paradigms, and goals, be used in nursing without modification? There are also questions that relate to the methods themselves. Are these methods simply techniques for data collection and analysis, or must they be used within the context of their discipline's theoretical assumptions and perspectives (Morse 1991)? Conceptual confusion is almost always present, extending beyond the methods themselves. For example, "phenomenology" may be used to refer to a philosophical stance, a qualitative research method, or to qualitative research in general. Another area of concern is the use of qualitative methods to test theory. Morse (1991) states: "The strength of qualitative methods is in the process of induction; the data 'emerge' to provide a theory, not the reverse. Qualitative data cannot be categorized to fit into a framework" (pp. 16–17). From these methodological concerns arising from the 1990s, questions still occur now in the twenty-first century. The questions that Morse (1991) asked are still applicable to this day: (i) Should qualitative methods be rigorously prescriptive, as are quantitative methods, or loosely described in order to give investigators the freedom to develop their own style? (ii) If the qualitative methods that originated from other disciplines must be adapted to nursing, who is responsible for this process of modification and is this a matter of trial and error? (p. 17).

2.1 Nature and Design of a Qualitative Phenomenological Study

A qualitative study begins with our posing a broad research question focusing on a phenomenon about which little is known (Cypress 2015). The process of designing a qualitative study begins *not* with the methods – which is actually the easiest part of the research – but with the broad assumption central to the inquiry. After a research question has been identified, the researcher needs a thorough understanding of the philosophical assumptions that are the foundation of the method. Almost always, novice researchers develop and conduct research studies beginning with the methods, without having a solid understanding of the philosophical underpinnings or the broad assumptions central to the qualitative inquiry. This lack of understanding has the potential to lead to sloppy science, resulting in misunderstood findings. Ironside (2005) argues that "the nature of inquiry is determined more by researchers' pre-given understandings than by the rules or guidelines detailing 'proper' methodological procedures for epistemological development. Methods are not directed to an end (an answer) but constantly self-renew as questioning continues" (p. xvi).

Among novice qualitative researchers, and even experts, confusion and uncertainty are evident around how to use the phenomenological approach, and the underpinning philosophical assumptions and paradigms or worldviews. The problem seems to reside in the fact that phenomenology is a philosophy, a foundation for qualitative research, as well as a research method in its own right (Eddles-Hirsch 2015). Adding to the dilemma is the fact that phenomenology is one not unified approach. It actually consists of three disparate complex philosophies – transcendental, existential, and existential-embodied – with their corresponding methodologies: descriptive, hermeneutic or interpretive, and descriptive-hermeneutic.

For a new naturalistic researcher planning to delve into a phenomenological study, it is easier to label the inquiry "qualitative phenomenological," especially if the research adviser has an inadequate background and training in philosophy and phenomenological research methodologies. This creates problems because not knowing whether a study is descriptive, hermeneutic/interpretive, or a combination of both leads to a faulty selection of methodological procedures and consequently questionable results. Thus, it is important for phenomenological researchers to identify and state early on the approach that they will adopt for their research (Eddles-Hirsch 2015). An expert qualitative researcher and phenomenologist with a good grasp of philosophy available to act as adviser or mentor is necessary to guide the new investigator on the difficult journey of doing a phenomenological investigation.

2.2 Paradigms and Worldviews

It is evident in the literature that there are misconceptions and confusion among qualitative nurse researchers about the meaning of "paradigm." Some mistakenly equate paradigm to either quantitative or qualitative methodology (Risjord 2010). Risjord (2010) asserts that there is a mismatch between the idea of a paradigm and the philosophical commitments of nursing researchers. He says the problem is the idea of a "quantitative and qualitative paradigm," and that both are associated to a *theory*. Nurses assume that any theory that is testable by measurements is supposed to be part of a quantitative paradigm, and that "qualitative" is associated with phenomenology. Risjord (2010) further expresses that "There is no quantitative paradigm because there is no single quantitative theory with ontological commitments, or implications for methodology. Here, the problem is not that there are too many theories; there are none at all. Phenomenology is not a theory in Kuhn's sense. It is a broad, and varied school of philosophical thought" (p. 200). Phenomenology has been beneficial to nursing as a body of methodological ideas that support the use of qualitative methods, but qualitative methodology is often difficult since it requires sensitive interpretive skills and creative talents on the part of the researcher (van Manen 2014). There is a need for some clarity on paradigms and qualitative phenomenological research.

In qualitative research, inquirers make assumptions. According to Creswell (2007), these philosophical assumptions consist of a stance toward the nature of reality (ontology), how the researchers know and what they know (epistemology), the role of values in research (axiology), the language of research (rhetoric), and the methods used in the process (methodology) (p. 16). Qualitative researchers take a philosophical stance on each of these assumptions when they decide to undertake a naturalistic inquiry. After they make their choice, the study is further shaped by the paradigms or worldviews that they bring to the research study.

A paradigm is a basic set of beliefs that guide action (Creswell 2007). It is impossible to conduct any type of investigation without committing to ontological and epistemological positions, which every paradigm is based upon. Paradigms present varying views, and researchers have differing assumptions, set of beliefs about reality, and pools of knowledge, as well as different positions toward a given phenomenon, which underpin their particular approach. This is reflected in their methodology and methods (Scotland 2012). A researcher can combine aspects of different paradigms and traditions. Since a paradigm's fundamental assumptions about the world determine what questions may (and may not) be asked, methodological choices only make sense in the context of a paradigm (Risjord 2010). It is important in a research design to make explicit what paradigm a researcher will work on. Using an established paradigm allows one to build on a coherent and well-developed approach to research (Maxwell 2005). Some examples of paradigms or worldviews are post-positivism, social constructivism, advocacy/participatory, and pragmatism (Creswell 2007). Table 2.1 lists different philosophical assumptions and the questions that researchers will ask before starting a qualitative study in each

Table 2.1 Philosophical assumptions and questions to ask.

Assumption	Question
Ontological	What is the nature of reality?
Epistemological	What is the relationship between the researcher and that being searched?
Axiological	What is the role of values?
Rhetorical	What is the language of research?
Methodological	What is the process of research?

Source: Creswell, J. W. (2007). Qualitative inquiry and research design: Choosing among five approaches, 2nd ed., Sage Publications.

case (Creswell 2007). Table 2.2 describes the assumptions and how they relate to the positions of the paradigms (Creswell 2007; Guba and Lincoln 1994). Table 2.3 describes the issues and positions of constructivism that have important impacts on the conduct of an inquiry (Creswell 2007; Guba and Lincoln 1994). The focus of this chapter is on social constructivism as it manifests in phenomenological studies.

Social constructivism is often combined with interpretivism. The goal of the research is to describe and understand the subjective meanings that individuals attach to the world in which they live and work, and it is negotiated socially and historically, allowing them numerous viewpoints on reality (not only one reality). This worldview manifests in phenomenological studies, in which individuals describe their *lived* experiences of a phenomenon. The researcher is an active participant and cannot be detached from the participant being studied. Phenomenologists use an emergent qualitative approach to inquiry, collect data in a natural setting from individuals who have experienced or lived the phenomenon, and analyze it in an inductive way until patterns or themes emerge and are illuminated. Any substantial prior structuring of the methods leads to a lack of flexibility to respond to emergent insights and can create methodological "tunnel vision" in making sense of the data (Creswell 2007). No preconceived theories or frameworks guide the collection and analysis of data. Theories, models, and explanations are not generated from the analysis (Morse 1991). Researchers also recognize that their own background shapes their interpretation and acknowledge how their interpretation flows from their own personal, cultural, and historical experiences (Creswell 2007). The final written report includes the voices of participants, the reflexivity of the researcher, and a complex description and interpretation of the phenomenon.

2.3 Phenomenology-as-Philosophy

Phenomenology has a strong philosophical component to it (Streubert and Carpenter 1999). From a philosophical viewpoint, the study of humans is deeply rooted in *descriptive* modes of science. Human scientists have been concerned with describing the fundamental patterns of human thought and behavior since early times (Streubert

Table 2.2 Paradigms and worldviews.

Assumptions	Post-positivism	Social Constructivism	Advocacy/ Participatory	Pragmatism
Ontology	Critical realism – real "reality" but only imperfectly and probabilistically apprehendable	Relativism (constructed realities); interpretivism	"Voice" of participants heard throughout the research process	Not committed to any one system or philosophy; external world independent of the mind; belief of not asking questions about reality and laws of nature; world is not an absolute unity
Epistemology	Modified dualist objectivist; reductionistic; critical tradition/community findings probably true	Transactional/ subjectivist; subjective meanings are negotiated socially and historically; focus is on specific contexts of people; addresses the processes of interaction among individuals; understanding of the world; created findings; researchers inductively develop a theory or pattern of meaning	Alternative view; contain an action agenda for reform that may change the lives of participants, researchers, and institutions	Truth is what works at the time; not based on dualism between reality independent of the mind or within the mind
Methodology	Modified experimental/ manipulative; critical multiplism; chiefly quantitative methods; falsification of hypothesis; emphasis on empirical data collection; cause-and-effect oriented; deterministic based on priori theories; may include qualitative methods	Hermeneutic/dialectical	Participatory action is recursive/ dialectical; emancipatory; practical; collaborative	Researchers are "free" and have the freedom of choice on methods and procedures of research; the "what" and "how" to research is based on its intended consequences – where they want to go with it rather than the antecedent conditions; methods are not the focus, rather the problem and questions being studied; may include mixed methods research

Sources: Based on Creswell, J. W. (2007). Qualitative inquiry and research design: Choosing among five approaches, 2nd ed., Sage Publications and Guba, E. G., & Lincoln, Y. S. (1994). Competing paradigms in qualitative research.

Table 2.3 Constructivism and paradigm position.

Issue	Constructivism
Inquiry aim	Understanding; reconstruction
Nature of knowledge	Individual reconstruction; coalescing around consensus
Knowledge accumulation	More informed and sophisticated; vicarious experience
Goodness and quality criteria	Trustworthiness and authenticity
Values	Included-formative
Ethics	Intrinsic; process tilt toward revelation
Voice	"Passionate" participant as facilitator of multi-voice reconstruction

Sources: Based on Creswell, J. W. (2007). Qualitative inquiry and research design: Choosing among five approaches, 2nd ed., Sage Publications and Guba, E. G., & Lincoln, Y. S. (1994). Competing paradigms in qualitative research.

and Carpenter 1999). For example, phenomenologists who support Edmund Husserl – the "father of phenomenology" – and his followers believe that the purpose of phenomenology is to provide pure understanding (descriptive phenomenology). The phenomenological tradition began with Husserl in the 1890s, when it was labeled *transcendentalism*. Sandelowski (2000) asserts that the qualitative descriptive study is the method of choice when straight descriptions of phenomena are desired, especially for researchers wanting to know the "who," "what," and "where" of events. It is a fact that, foundational to all qualitative research approaches, qualitative descriptive studies represent a valuable methodologic approach in and of themselves. Sandelowski (2000) further articulates that "If [phenomonologists'] studies were designed with overtones from other methods, they can describe what these overtones were, instead of inappropriately naming or implementing these other methods" (p. 339). On the opposite pole, supporters of the philosophical positions of Martin Heidegger and his colleagues believe that phenomenology is *interpretive or hermeneutic,* and *existential.* Neither approach (descriptive and hermeneutic/interpretive) is incorrect. Each comes to the study of lived experiences with different perspectives, sets of goals, and expectations. From Husserl, Merleau-Ponty (1945/1962) suggests that phenomenology is a philosophy that sees people in a world that already exists before any reflection. He sees the individual as the body itself, at a place and time, acting in the world in which it lives. He combines Husserl's transcendental approach to epistemological questions with an existential orientation derived from Heidegger. Merleau-Ponty's philosophical approach is referred to as *existential-embodied.*

2.3.1 Edmund Husserl's Transcendental Philosophy

Husserl is often called "the founder of phenomenology." Drawing from his background in mathematics, psychology, and Kantian philosophy, he defined phenomenology as the systematic study of the essential content of our experiences that is epistemological and pure or *transcendental* (Husserl 1973, 1983). Epistemology is the branch of philosophy concerned with the nature and grounds of knowledge. He espoused for realism – a realism that is very distant from the naïve realism of the "natural attitude," or the empiricism of the hard sciences (Tarozzi and Mortari 2010). He advocated a departure from science and claims that experience is the fundamental source of knowledge and some important features of experiences are subjectively constituted. For Husserl, phenomenology was the rigorous and unbiased study of things as they appear, in order to arrive at an essential understanding of human consciousness and experience. He believed that by using the transcendental reduction process, one could delve deeply into consciousness and uncover the underlying structures of a phenomenon. His philosophy is descriptive in that pre-reflective experiences should be careful, elaborate descriptions that focus on *essences* rather than concepts or facts, which can change over time or between cultural contexts (Kaufer and Chemero 2015). Phenomenology as discussed by Husserl (1983) is a return to the lifeworld – the world of experience. The idea of the lifeworld refers to the pre-reflexive or pre-objective world that should be understood without resorting to interpretations. Husserl asserted that there is a phenomenon only when there is a subject who experiences that phenomenon. Husserl emphasized that a phenomenon should be described instead of explained or interpreted. He criticized positivism, and emphasized that the causal relations of phenomena should not be searched for, that the focus should be on the very things as they manifest themselves.

2.3.1.1 Intentionality

Intentionality, according to Husserl, is the basic characteristic of phenomena and the core of phenomenology. It is also the most important feature of consciousness. Intentional acts are immanent, mind-internal, and given to us completely. Our consciousness is oriented externally to the things and experience of the world. Through the intentionality of consciousness, all actions, gestures, and habits (human and otherwise) have meaning. All meaningful experiences occur in acts, and all conscious acts are unified and transparent. Consciousness, through such intentionality, is understood as the agent that attributes meanings to objects. Without these meanings, it would be impossible to talk either about an object or about an object's essence (Kaufer and Chemero 2015; Sadala and Adorno 2002).

2.3.1.2 Epoché and Eidetic Reduction

Husserl (1981) presents *epoché* and *reduction* as key elements of phenomenology. He developed the method of epoché, or "bracketing," around 1906. Epoché is a Greek word that means "to refrain from judgment, or to stay away from everyday common place of perceiving things" (Moustakas 1994). It refers to a non-conditioned attitude that is sufficiently open, available to listen, unbiased, and non-judging (Tarozzi and Mortari 2010). Epoché, together with eidetic reduction, forms the essential core of the transcendental-phenomenological method introduced in *Ideas* (Husserl 1983). It has us focus on those aspects of our intentional acts and their contents that do not depend on the existence of a represented object out there in the extra-mental world. Thus, epoché is one means to achieve reduction (Husserl 1973, 1983). Reduction, according to Husserl, involves taking the world as it is considered in the natural attitude and reducing it to a world of pure phenomena – or, more poetically, to a purely phenomenal realm. In the *natural attitude*, individuals hold knowledge judgmentally (Dowling 2007; Moustakas 1994). Tarozzi and Mortari (2010) state: "For phenomenologists, the *epoché* not only reminds us that we are always embedded in our prejudices and pre-comprehensions, so that we should distance ourselves from them, and suspend judgment about them, but represents first and foremost a transition that introduces us to a cognitive and heuristic path of reduction" (p. 28). Reductions can be either *eidetic* or *transcendental*. In either case, they are called *phenomenological reduction* (Husserl 1981; Kaufer and Chemero 2015).

Eidetic reduction is the shifting of focus from accidental or non-essential features of an experience to essential ones, keeping only the essence of the phenomenon under study. Transcendental reduction is the shifting of focus from the object of experience to the way that the object is constituted (Kaufer and Chemero 2015). Phenomenological reduction is the fundamental resource that ensures a reliable description of a phenomenon, brackets the reality conceived by common sense, and cleanses the phenomenon of everything that is "unessential" and accidental in order to make what is essential visible (Husserl 1981; Sadala and Adorno 2002). Thus, a researcher should maintain a phenomenological stance by avoiding any judgment from interfering with their openness to the description, should set aside any prior thought and conception that they may have about the phenomenon (epoché). The focus is on the *essence* and description of the phenomenon in its specific context. The essence is the very nature of what is being questioned (Sadala and Adorno 2002).

2.3.2 Martin Heidegger's Existential Philosophy

Martin Heidegger was a student and assistant of Husserl. His work was influenced by Dilthey (1985), focusing on *interpretation*, and Soren Kierkegaard's *existentialism* (Solomon 1974). Heidegger's phenomenological philosophy is existential and hermeneutic (Heidegger 1992). He was destined to reject Husserl's (1983) understanding that phenomenology is the science of essences. Rather than exploration and description of experiences, he advocated for the utilization of hermeneutics as a research method founded on the ontological view that lived experience is an *interpretive* process (Dowling 2007; Heidegger 1992).

Heidegger's conception of phenomenology departs from the Husserlian mode of analysis of consciousness. In his book *Being and Time* (Heidegger 1927/1962), he proposes that consciousness is not separate from the world of human existence. For him, phenomenology is a method of philosophy that is ontological, and its primary phenomenon is the meaning of *being* (presence in the world). Ontology is the branch of philosophy that is about the nature of being. To ask for the being of something is to ask for the nature or meaning of that phenomenon. *Being-in-the-world* refers to the way humans exist, act, or are involved in the world (Dowling 2007; van Manen 1990), or the to the notion that knowledge of our everyday existence is intersubjective, temporal, and relational (Evans and O'Brien 2005). Phenomenology grounded in the Heideggerian tradition represents a shift from an epistemological emphasis on an understanding of essences and the seeking of universal truths to an existential-ontological understanding of a person's being-in-the-world (Evans and O'Brien 2005). While Husserl emphasized understanding of individual experience through bracketing, Heidegger believed that it was impossible to set aside one's own presuppositions and beliefs. He asserted that intrinsic awareness is fundamental to phenomenological research, as the researcher needs to be immersed within the phenomenon to gain an understanding of the experience (Eddles-Hirsch 2015). Nurse researchers such as Benner and Wrubel (1989) adopted Heideggerian philosophy in their study of caring in nursing, while Walsh (1999) used it in her research into nurse–patient encounters in psychiatric care.

2.3.3 Merleau-Ponty's Existential-Embodied Philosophy

Merleau-Ponty (1945/1962) built on the writings of Husserl and Heidegger. He suggested that phenomenology is the rigorous science of the search for essences. He combined Husserl's transcendental approach to epistemological questions with an existential orientation derived from Heidegger. The specific aim of his phenomenology was to give direct description, not a causal explanation of experience. Lived experience given in the perceived world must be described (Merleau-Ponty 1956). Merleau-Ponty also emphasized that phenomenology is a philosophy that sees people in a world that already exists before any reflection. He saw the individual as the body itself, at a place and time, acting in the world in which it lived. The body itself is the perceiving subject: the point of view of the world, the time–space structure of the perceiving experience. Merleau-Ponty proposed the task of returning to the very thing in a search for the essences of objects, their qualities – but saw these as part of the lived and experienced world, which is a world of things that have not been reflected upon, and on which sciences are constructed. He believed that it is through the life experience that a person has the potential to find meaning and understanding in life.

Merleau-Ponty (1945/1962) argued that the lived body was not an object in the world, but rather the person's point of view of the world. The body itself is the knowing object. He was concerned with a science of human being, and that the relation between human and world was ontological. Merleau-Ponty (1945/1962) stated: "It is through my relation to others, and also through my relation to things that I know myself" (p. 383). Further, he emphasized that intentionality is relatedness to the world, the integral connectedness between humans and the lifeworld in which human attention is always directed toward specific events, objects, and phenomena. For Merleau-Ponty (1964), in this condition of being in a situation in an already given world of relationships, the other's universality leads them to a selective operation in order to adapt to the situation. Each body, with its own structure, selects ways to adapt, which are never repeated either with others or with itself at other moments and places. Understanding the meaning of some experience requires us to describe the intentional stance (or situated perspective) of the event from the point of view of the experiencing person. This is also related to his concept of relationality.

Merleau-Ponty's phenomenological philosophy has been useful to nurse researchers for many years. This is evident in the utilization of the four existentials considered to belong to the fundamental structure of the lifeworld – lived space (spatiality), lived body (corporeality), lived time (temporality), and lived human relation (relationality or communality) – which are productive for the process of phenomenological questioning, reflecting, and writing (van Manen 1990).

2.3.3.1 Exemplar: Using Merleau-Ponty's Phenomenological Philosophy in Understanding the Lived Experiences of Patients, Family Members, and their Nurses During Critical Illness in the Intensive Care Unit

Phenomenological research begins with wonder at what gives itself and how something gives itself. Surrendering to such a state of wonder gives way to a phenomenon. A phenomenon is an event or a lived-through experience as it shows itself or as it gives itself when it makes an appearance in our awareness. It does not manifest itself because of human willing, but occurs as we deal with it (van Manen 2014). The phenomenon of interest for this phenomenological study is the lived experiences of patients, family members, and their nurses during critical illness in the intensive care unit (**ICU**). How does one decide to use the phenomenological approach for a topic needing investigation? What phenomena important to nursing lend themselves to this type of qualitative inquiry? The answers to these questions are grounded in philosophical beliefs about humans and the holistic nature of professional nursing. Investigation of phenomena vital to nursing requires that researchers study lived experiences as they are presented in the everyday world of nursing practice. The phenomenological approach supports new initiatives for nursing care where the subject matter is often not amenable to other investigative and experimental methods.

2.3.3.1.1 Prologue I was a critical care nurse for 20 years. As I reflect on my long experience, I can say that caring for the critically ill brought meaning to my life related to the knowledge and experiences I gained from such a career in nursing. I have continuously engaged in providing care to critically ill patients with varied, multiple acute conditions and their families in a diversity of critical care settings. I have seen patients who, after a critical illness, recovered fully or with positive outcomes, and those with poor outcomes resulting in disability and even death. I noticed that there were an increasing number of patients with prolonged length of stay in the ICU related to complications, co-morbidities, and exacerbation of chronic health illnesses. As the phenomenon became clearer to me, I asked the questions, "Is there a need for further clarity on this phenomenon of interest?" and, "Is there anything published on this subject, or does what is published need to be described in more depth?" My positive response to both these questions helped clarify that the phenomenological approach is the most appropriate for the study. Past studies have examined the effects of critical illness on both the patient and their family members, including the nurses' ICU experiences. These studies were done either from the perspectives of nurses, patients, and family members individually or from that between nurse and patient, nurse and family, and patient and family. There is a scarcity of research studies in the literature conducted on the triad of nurses, patients, and family members looking at the experience of critical illness and the perspectives of one relating to the others. Most of the studies related to critical illness and families are also quantitative, with a focus on selected areas of concern or selected individuals in the family. Studies that describe the experiences of the triad of nurses, patients, and family members during critical illness in the ICU reveal a gap in the literature that is left unexplored, and one that I seek to fill. By conducting this phenomenological research, I aim to further explore, describe, understand, and illuminate the meaning of ICU experience as perceived by patients, their family members, and their nurses.

Phenomenological inquiry requires that the integrated whole be explored, thus it is a suitable approach for this phenomenon important to nursing practice. Phenomenology also aims to describe phenomena in rich language as they present themselves. It is more a method of questioning than of answering, with the realization that insights come to us in the modes of musing, reflective questioning, and being obsessed with the sources and meanings of lived experiences. By understanding the meaning of ICU experience from the perspective of the three key players, I hope to contribute knowledge that could impact the provision of care in the ICU, thus improving patient outcomes. After the phenomenon of interest has been explicitly identified and the purpose of the study has been clearly delineated, research questions will be posed.

A phenomenological question explores what is given in moments of pre-reflective, pre-predicative experience as we live through them. The research questions that guide this study are: (i) What are the patients' and their families' experiences of the nurse in an ICU environment? and (ii) What are the nurses' experiences of the patients and families in an ICU environment? Once these research questions are posed, philosophical assumptions are made that help guide methodological decisions and a well-developed phenomenological research design. The philosophical perspective of Merleau-Ponty (1945/1962) is used for this exemplary study.

Merleau-Ponty (1945/1962) suggests that phenomenology is the study of essences – the essence of perception or consciousness. This is a philosophy that puts essences back into existence and does not expect to arrive at an understanding of humanity and the world from any starting point other than that of their facticity (p. vii). Merleau-Ponty (1945/1962) asserts that phenomenology shall be a rigorous science, but it also offers an account of space, time, and the world as we "live" them. The lived body is not an object in the world but rather the person's point of view of the world. He is concerned with a science of human being, and that the relation between human and world is ontological. The specific aim of his phenomenology is to give a direct description, not a causal explanation of experience. Lived experience given in the perceived world must be described, not constructed or formed.

Merleau-Ponty (1945/1962) proposes the task of returning to the very thing in a search for the essences of objects, their qualities – but seeing these as part of the lived and experienced world, which is a world of things that have not been reflected upon and on which sciences are constructed. This means that one cannot put perception into the same category as the syntheses represented by judgments, acts, or predication (p. xi). Perception is not a science of the world, it is not even an act, a deliberate taking up of a position; it is the background from which all acts stand out, and is presupposed by them (p. xi). Merleau-Ponty states: "When I return to myself from an excursion into the realm of dogmatic common sense of science, I find not a source of intrinsic truth, but a subject destined to the world" (p. xii) . . . "The world is not what I think but what I live through" (p. xviiii). The phenomenological world is not the bringing to explicit expression of a pre-existing being, but the laying down of being, and such phenomenology is only accessible through a phenomenological method (p. viii). Phenomenology, as a disclosure of the world, rests on itself, and its task is to reveal the mystery of the world and of reason.

After developing an overall phenomenological approach and determining a philosophical perspective, considerations for sampling decisions, data collection, analysis, and interpretation are made. Qualitative research designs are not fixed and static; rather, they are emergent and flexible. In qualitative studies, sampling, data collection, and analysis – including interpretation – take place repetitively. Informed consent is also an ongoing process that continues until data saturation is achieved (process consent). The sampling method usually used is purposive.

A purposeful sample of five nurses, five patients, and five family members in the ICU is included. The patient participants in this study are acutely, critically ill patients in the ICU prior to transfer to the regular medical floor, with age ranging from 22 to 70 years. Eligibility is determined to ensure the patients' mental capabilities to answer questions and tell their stories, keeping in mind per Merleau-Ponty (1945/1962) that "To remember is not to bring into the focus of consciousness a self-subsistent picture of the past; it is to trust deeply into the horizon of the past and take apart step-by-step the interlocked perspectives until the experiences which it epitomizes are as if relived in their temporal setting. To perceive is not to remember" (p. 26). All the nurses participating in this study hold a bachelor of science in nursing, are registered nurses in New York State, are aged between 25 and 60 years, and have at least two years of critical care experience in the ICU. The sample of family members includes patients' spouses, a daughter, and a patient's mother, all of whom spend a great deal of time at the bedside in the ICU and are aged between 22 and 70 years old. These family members are the patients' immediate family, significant others, primary support systems, and caregivers, and are named by patients as their family.

Rigorous data collection procedures occurred over six months, comprising in-depth face-to-face interviews, in order to explore the phenomenon under study. An inductive approach to data analysis was taken. Data analysis began with the very first data collection, to facilitate the emergent design and structure. Analysis of the data proceeded with a description of the lived experiences of all 15 participants of critical illness in the ICU and with an interpretation of the overall meaning of the individual interviews. The transcripts were approached with an open attitude, seeking what emerged as important and of interest from the texts. The understanding of a thing written is not a repetition of something past but the sharing of a present meaning. No conceptual or single statements can capture the full mystery of the ICU experience of the participants. Merleau-Ponty (1945/1962) states: "The act of understanding presents itself as reflection on an unreflective experience which it does not absorb either in fact or in theory . . . Reflection never lifts itself out of any situation, nor does the analysis of perception do away with the fact of perception, the thisness of the percept or the inherence of perceptual consciousness in some temporality, and some locality. Reflection in not absolutely transparent for itself . . . Between the self which analyzes perception and the self which perceives, there is always a distance" (p. 49). A thematic phrase does not do justice to the fullness of the life of a phenomenon. It only serves to point, to allude, or to hint at an aspect of a phenomenon. These processes and considerations facilitated the articulation of structural patterns related to the perceived ICU experiences across all participant interviews' texts.

Phenomenology as an approach for my study allowed the description and under-standing of the phenomenon of interest. Merleau-Ponty (1945/1962) states: "The description of phenomena does not enable one to refute thought which is not alive to its own existence, and which resides in things" (p. 26). Themes were first generally classified into two categories: the integrating common themes and the specific themes. A total of five integrating common themes were illuminated. The lived ICU experience among all the participants is interdependence. The patients, their family members, and their nurses are one or intertwined. Adaptation in the ICU, as experienced by the participants from three categories, integrates family as a unit, physical care/comfort, physiological care, and psychosocial support resulting in transformation. The second set of themes was categorized into nurse-specific, patient-specific, and family members-specific. A total of three themes were illuminated: (i) advocacy; (ii) uncertainty; and (iii) confidence in the nurse and healthcare team. These themes constituted the essential essences of the perceived experience of the nurses of patients and family members and of the patients and families of the nurses in the study. The findings are further discussed from the philosophical perspective of Merleau-Ponty (1945/1962).

Merleau-Ponty's (1945/1962) existentials of embodiment, relationality, spatiality, and temporality belong to the fundamental structure of the lifeworld – the world of lived experience in which humans experience the world, but not in the same modality. We all experience our world and our reality through these existentials. Embodiment, spatiality, temporality, and relationality are productive categories for the process of phenomenological question posing, reflecting, and writing (van Manen 1990, 2014).

2.3.3.1.2 The Critically Ill Patient and Lived Body (Embodiment) The existential theme of embodiment (lived body) may guide our reflection as to how the body is experienced based on the phenomenon that is being studied. Some phenomeno-logical authors regard body and embodiment as the fundamental motif of their under-standing of human phenomena. Merleau-Ponty (1945/1962) is the phenomenologist of the body (van Manen 2014). He states: "The body is the vehicle of being in the world, and having a body is, for a living creature, to be intervolved in a definite environment" (p. 94) . . . "To be a body, is to be tied to a certain world . . . our body is not primarily in space" (p. 171) . . . "It is as much of my essence to have a body as it is the future's to be the future of certain present . . . It is not only the notion of the body which through that of the present, it is necessarily linked to that of the for-itself; the actual existence of my body is indispensable to that of my consciousness" (p. 501). Further: "The body and the mind communicate with each other through the medium of time, that to be a mind is to stand above time's flow and to have a body is to have a present" (p. 91) . . . "It is by abandoning the body as an object, *partes extra partes,* and by going back to the body which I experience at this moment . . . I cannot understand the function of the living body except by enacting it myself, and except in so far as I am a body which rises towards the world" (p. 87).

Merleau-Ponty (1945/1962) emphasizes the sacredness of the body and explained that when the relationship between body and world is disturbed (i.e., when bodily capacities are changed related to critical illness), a person's existence is shaken. A change in the body and in physical and perceptual possibility transforms subjectivity itself. The lived experiences of critically ill patients in the ICU relates to Merleau-Ponty's discussion of the phantom limb, in which he states: "I am conscious of the world through my body. It is precisely when my customary world arouses me in habitual intentions that I can no longer, if I have lost a limb, be effectively drawn into it, and the utilizable objects . . . appeal to a hand which I no longer have. Thus are delimited, in the totality of my body, regions of silence . . . Our body comprises as it were two distinct layers, that of the *habit-body* and that of the *body this moment* . . . How can the habitual body act as guarantee for the body at this moment? How can I perceive objects as manipulatable if I can no longer manipulate them? The manipulatable must have ceased to be what I am now manipulating, and become what one can manipulate; it must have ceased to be a thing *manipulatable for me* and become a thing *manipulatable in itself*. Correspondingly, my body must be apprehended not only in an experience which is instantaneous, peculiar to itself and complete in itself, but also in some general aspect and in the light of impersonal being" (p. 95). In this study, the patient's embodiment (habit-body) is threatened by critical illness, which has effects and meanings for their lifeworld and lived experience. Critical illness is a life-threatening disease or state in which death is possible or imminent, affecting both the patient and their family members. Shem (1978) provides an array of descriptions of critical illness in intensive care:

> *Just as Jo, the head nurse, and I were wheeling the chart rack to the first room, in skipped Pinkus, the Consultant to the unit, ready to start his teaching rounds . . . Of the other five patients, none could speak. Each suffered in the throes of some horrible, incurable, lingering disease that would almost certainly kill usually involving major organs like heart, lung, liver, kidney, and the brain. The most pathetic was a man who had started with a pimple on his knee . . . I saw his eyes fasten on me, a newcomer, someone who might bring a miracle, asking me to give him back his voice, his Saturday afternoon game of squash, his piggyback rides under his kids . . . I turned my head away. I never wanted to look into those mute eyes again.*
>
> *He was not alone. Four more times I was shaken by the horror of ruined life. One after the other, totally immobilized, lungs run by respirators, heart run by pacemakers, kidneys run by machines, brains run barely, if at all. It was terrible. The smell was that of lingering death . . . I left. As I drove through the chill April rain, my mind stuck on the unit. What about it had been so different?*
>
> *Quintessence. That was it. The unit was the quintessence. There after all the sorting had been done; lay the closest representation, in living terms, of death . . . Berry asked me how it had been, and I told her that it had been different, high-powered, kind of like being part of the manned space program, but it was also like being in a vegetable garden, only the vegetables were human. (pp. 324–330)*

This description provides only a glimpse of the critical care world. It is a place where the patient's life-threatening processes are treated, and where life and health situations transpire recurrently. For Merleau-Ponty (1945/1962), "in cases of illness, the bodily events become the events of the day. What enables us to centre our existence is also what prevents us from centring it completely, and the anonymity of our body is inseparably both freedom and servitude. Thus, to sum up, the ambiguity of being-in-the-world is translated by that of the body, and is understood through that of time" (p. 98) . . . "Time in its passage does not carry away with it these impossible projects; it does not close up on traumatic experience; the subject (critically ill patient) remains open to the same impossible future, if not in his explicit thoughts, at any rate in his actual being . . . it displaces the others and deprives them of their value as authentic presents . . . Impersonal time continues its course, but personal time is arrested" (p. 69) . . . "To the extent that I have 'sense organs,' a body, and psychic functions comparable with other men's, each of the moments of my experience ceases to be an integrated and strictly unique totality, in which details exist only in virtue of the whole, I become the host of 'causalities' . . . a margin of almost impersonal existence which can be practically taken for granted . . . personal existence represses the organism without being able to either go beyond it or to renounce itself; without in other words, being able to reduce the organism to its existential self, or itself to the organism . . . Personal existence is intermittent, and when this tide turns and recedes, decision can henceforth endow my life with only an artificially induced significance. The fusion of the soul and body in the act, the sublimation of biological into personal existence is made possible and precarious by the temporal structure of our experience" (pp. 96–97).

The term "critical care unit" involves images of very ill patients surrounded by the latest in biomedical equipment, noisy monitoring devices, and emergency carts. These images, along with the level of technology and equipment in the ICU environment, raise feelings of anxiety and levels of stress in patients and families alike (Farrell et al. 2005). The ICU is a foreign place where everything appears bizarre, from the critical nature of admission to the strange environment, unfamiliar caregivers, and obscure language. There is a plethora of unfamiliar sounds, smells, and sights. Thus, the ICU creates a stressful environment. Intensive care also serves the most acutely ill of hospital patients, or those with critical illnesses. According to Zussman (1992), intensive care is not a technology, it is a place in which technology is applied daily to the most intractable of medical problems. Most generally, the principal roles of intensive care are life-support of organ system failure in critically-ill patients and close monitoring of stable, non-critically-ill patients in case the need for life support suddenly occurs (body that is *manipulatable in itself*). Zussman (1992) further states: "Perhaps Lazarus is not quite raised from the dead but it is in intensive care that the miracles of modern medical technology are reenacted routinely and methodically" (p. 21). The existential theme of *spatiality* may guide our reflection to ask how space (ICU) is experienced related to the phenomenon of this study.

2.3.3.1.3 The Critically Ill Patient and Lived Space (Spatiality)
Merleau-Ponty (1945/1962) asserts that our bodies occupy a space: "Spatiality or lived space is felt space. Bodily spatiality is the deployment of one's bodily being, the way in which

the body comes into being as a body" (p. 172) . . . "The body can co-exist with the world. The constitution of a spatial level is simply one means of constituting an integrated world; my body is geared unto the world when my perception presents me with a spectacle . . . as they unfold receive the responses they expect from the world" (p. 292). It is our situatedness in the world that enables our reflection upon a past and gives a sense of past and future as parts of a bodily life. In this condition of being in a situation in an already given world of relationships, the other's universality leads them to a selective operation in order to adapt to the situation. Each body, with its own structure, selects ways to adapt, which are never repeated either with others or with themselves at other moments and places. Further, "It is a fact that I believe myself to be first of all surrounded by my body, involved in the world, situated here and now, but each of these words, when I come to think about them, is devoid of meaning, and therefore raises no problem: would I perceive myself as surrounded by my body if I were not in it as well as being in myself, if I did not myself conceive this spatial relationship and thus escape inherence at the very instant at which I conceive it? Would I know that I am caught up in the world? I should then merely be where I was, as a thing, and since I know where I am and see myself among things, it is because I am a consciousness, a strange creature which resides nowhere and can be everywhere present in intention" (p. 43). Understanding the meaning of some experience requires us to describe the intentional stance (or situated perspective) of the event from the point of view of the experiencing person. Space is existential (p. 342). This existential skill of situatedness and dwelling in the lifeworld enables a person to experience life as meaningful even in the face of illness (i.e., critical illness). But how is the space (ICU) experienced differently from place (home)? In what ways does the ICU environment affect the patient and their family members? How does the ICU space shape the patients and their families? The perception of a body implies the ability to change and to "understand" space (pp. 293–294). Further, Merleau-Ponty (1945/1962) states: "The shrinkage of lived space . . . leaves no room for chance. Like space, causality, before being a relation between objects, is based on my relation to things . . . Clear space, that impartial space in which all objects are equally important and enjoy the same right to existence, is not only surrounded, but also thoroughly permeated by another spatiality thrown into relief by morbid deviations from normal . . . he feels a threat hanging over him . . . Meanwhile, says the patient, 'a question is constantly put to me; it is as it were, an order either to rest or die, or else to push on further'" (p. 335). This second space, which cuts across visible space, is the one that is ceaselessly composed by our own way of projecting the world. Merleau-Ponty's example of a schizophrenic patient is like the ICU patient who no longer inhabits the common property world, but rather exists in the private world, and no longer gets as far as geographical space, but dwells in the "landscape space"; the landscape itself, once cut off from the common property world, is considerably impoverished; the patient's anguish, joy, and pain are related to a locality in objective space in which their empirical conditions are to be found (p. 336).

A patient who is confined to bed and on extensive monitoring often experiences discomforts, including pain. Sounds and lights from equipment in the ICU affect sleep, leading to perceptual deprivation and overload. Lusardi et al. (2011) report that the ICU is a dichotomy: high technology versus high touch, object versus subject, disease process versus personhood, and experience versus relation. It represents a concentration of the highest technological advances in the treatment and cure of life-threatening disease processes. On the one hand, it is a place of machinery such as ventilators, pacemakers, dialysis machines, and monitors, which assess and sustain life processes, and of disease processes and instabilities, which demand great attention and technical experience from the medical house staff. On the other, it is a place where humans with names and personhood come to survive life-threatening processes. In this phenomenological study, the patient's lived space is the ICU. The ICU is not the patient's usual environment. Critically ill patients in a high-technology environment such as the ICU experience a threat to their lived space as well as their physical and physiological being. Study participants perceived that physical care and comfort, coupled with physiological care, was vital during critical illness in the ICU. They identified bathing the patient, oral care, encouraging touch, treating the pain, and ensuring that the patient's room was clean as ways of providing physical care to the critically ill. In addition to taking vital signs, all participants identified giving medications and feeding patients as other ways of providing physiological care.

2.3.3.1.4 The Critically Ill Patient and Lived Time (Temporality) Merleau-Ponty (1945/1962) asserts that our embodied bodies occupy a space, and that space is located in time (temporality). Space is an aspect of time, and time is an aspect of space. Time is not a real process. It arises from one's relation to things (p. 478). Time is thought by us before its parts and temporal relations make possible the events in time (p. 481). The existential theme of *temporality* (lived time) may guide our reflection in asking how time is experienced relative to the lived experiences of patients and family members during critical illness in the ICU. How does the critically ill patient experience the passing of time and their *being* in the ICU? Do ICU patients even have a sense of time when they are critically ill? Time in our primordial experience of it is not for us a system of objective positions, through which we pass, but a mobile setting that moves away from us (p. 487). Since, in time, being and passing are synonymous, by becoming past, the event does not cease to be. Time maintains what it has caused to be at the very time, while its fixed position lying beneath our gaze is not to be sought in any eternal synthesis, but in the mutual harmonizing and overlapping of past and future through the present, and in the very passing of time. Temporality temporalizes itself as future, which lapses into the past by coming into the present (p. 488). We must understand time as the subject and the subject as time (p. 490). This primordial temporality is not a juxtaposition of external events, since it is the power that holds them together while keeping them apart.

Critically ill patients in ICU who are not awake, alert, and oriented (to person, place, and time) relative to sedation, chemically-induced coma, and paralysis have no concept of time. Days, weeks, or even months go by with the patient not knowing the date or whether it is night or day. Merleau-Ponty states: "What does not pass in time is the passing of time itself . . . Time restarts itself: the rhythmic cycle and constant form of yesterday, today and tomorrow . . . as the fountain creates in us a feeling of eternity" (p. 492). Critically ill patients may feel their suffering is never-ending: "The temporal perspective with its confusion of what is far removed in time, and that sort of 'shrinkage' of the past with oblivion as its ultimate limit, are not accidents of memory, and do not express the debasement into empirical existence of a consciousness of time theoretically all-embracing but its initial ambiguity: to retain is to hold but at a distance" (p. 491). Patients also have no sense of when they will recover from the critical illness, or whether they will recover at all. This begs the question, "Do critically ill patients come back in this way to a kind of eternity?" Eternity feeds on time. Merleau-Ponty further states: "I belong to my past, and through the constant interlocking of retentions, I preserve my oldest experiences, which means not duplicates or image of them, but the experiences themselves, exactly as they were. But the unbroken chain of the fields of presence, by which I am guaranteed access to the past itself, has the essential characteristic of being formed only gradually and one step at a time; each present in virtue of its very essence as a present, rules out the juxtaposition of other presents and, even in the context of a long time past" (p. 491). Death is also a common outcome of fatal and complicated illnesses. Critical illness is usually characterized by an acute incident that can be triggered by co-morbidities, which can lead to multiple admissions related to exacerbations, and ultimately chronicity. Patients are sometimes admitted in the ICU multiple times. They have little knowledge of when, how, or whether they will return to familiar surroundings (Lusardi et al. 2011). Further, Merleau-Ponty says, "It is of the essence of time to be not only actual time, or time which flows, but also time which is aware of itself. For the explosion or dehiscence of the present towards a future is the archetype of the relationship of self to self, and it traces out an inferiority" (p. 495).

Merleau-Ponty's (1945/1962) existentials of corporeality, spatiality, and temporality have been presented, but there are still questions that remain to be answered about the makeup of the person who is critically ill. Is it only the lived body, lived time, and lived space that are affected? How is the self experienced in relation to critical illness? Are family members affected? In what ways are the critically ill patient and their family members constituted? What is the role of the nurse in this equation? In what ways are the patient, their family members, and their nurses constituted?

2.3.3.1.5 The Critically Ill Patient and Lived Relation (Relationality)

The existential theme of *relationality* may guide our reflection to ask how self and others are experienced relative to the phenomenon of lived experiences of patients, family members, and nurses during critical illness in the ICU. Merleau-Ponty (1945/1962) states: "It is through my relation to others, and through my relation to things that I know myself" (p. 383) . . . "*I am given*, that is, I find myself already situated and involved in physical and social world . . . The physical and social world always function as a stimulus to my reactions, whether these be positive or negative" (pp. 419–420) . . . "We must therefore rediscover, after the natural world, the social world, not as an object or sum of objects, but a permanent field or dimension of existence . . . Our relationship to the social is, like our relationship to the world, deeper than any express perception or any judgement . . . We must return to the social with which we are in contact by the mere fact of existing, and which we carry about inseparably with us before any objectification. Objective and scientific consciousness of the past and civilizations would be impossible had I not, through the intermediary of my society, my cultural world and their horizons . . . The social is already there when we come to know or judge it" (pp. 421–422).

Simply, relationality refers to the fact that we always already find ourselves in a world and in relation to others.

Merleau-Ponty (1945/1962) believes in the benefits of connecting and relating with other people, and sees the potential for dialogue, through which persons receive recognition and affirmation. Life is spent in a "knot" or network of relations. He does not see others as impediments, but rather as fellow travelers in life's journey. Further, he states: "I am necessarily destined never to live through the presence of another to himself. And yet each other person does exist for me as an unchallengeable style or setting of co-existence and my life has a social atmosphere just as it has a flavor of mortality" (p. 425). Critical illness is a state of "inability" on the patient's part. Patients who are mechanically ventilated are unable to do certain things, perform certain roles, engage in certain activities, and consequently experience feelings of uncertainty, anxiety, panic, discomfort, loss of communication, insecurity, time disorientation, and altered self-image. Their family members are overwhelmed with feelings of fear, anxiety, and stress. Interactions with family, friends, and fellow workers are suspended and distorted. Critical illness may also lead to changes in the patient's support systems. Their experiences as they relate to finding meaning during critical illness center on obtaining support from their families and professionalism from their nurses. In this study, lived relation during the ICU experience was with their critically ill loved one, with each other, with nurses, physicians, and other healthcare staff, and with others who supported them. There is an implicit connection between physicians, nurses, family members, and healthcare staff and the ICU works as a whole because of this interdependence. To achieve relational integrity and effective adaptation during critical illness, patients must interact with their nurse, family members, and significant others for care, support, and security. ICU nurses are positioned to focus on caring for the patient. In order to provide holistic care, however, caring cannot be directed exclusively to the patient, especially in the context of critical illness. Care of the patient and family become intertwined, in that what affects one member potentially impacts the entire family. Thus, the hospitalization of a family member has an impact on the whole family system's equilibrium. To be able to help the family function in crisis related to critical illness, the nurse needs to promote adaptation and emotional stability.

The ICU experience among all the participants is interdependence. Interdependence is promoted by providing psychosocial support to patients and family members. Communication is identified as the precursor to providing psychosocial support. The descriptors for psychosocial support include emotional support, which includes encouragement, spiritual support, sensitivity to patients' and family members' needs, respect for the patient and family members, and the offering of translation services and referrals to social service. The patient, their family members, and their nurses are one, or intertwined. Nurses perceive patients and family members as a unit, and consequently patients and family members consider nurses as part of the family. There are three descriptors for this theme: involve the family in the plan of care or as an active participant; allow the family to bring pictures of the patient; and empathize with the family.

The meaning or essence of a phenomenon is never simple or one-dimensional. Meaning is multi-dimensional and multi-layered. Meaning never is and never can be finally complete. There is no end to meanings. They are infinite, always contextual, and recognized as expandable and expanding. Meaning is limited only by our unreadiness to enhance our understanding. The threat of possible researcher bias needs also to be considered.

Researcher bias is frequently an issue because qualitative research is open, exploratory, and less structured compared to quantitative research. It was important that I identified that my interest was not infused with bias and prejudice. Through reflexivity and bracketing, I was always on guard against my own biases, assumptions, beliefs, and presuppositions – but I was also aware that complete reduction is not possible. Van Manen (1990) notes that "If we simply try to forget or ignore what we already know, we may find that the presuppositions persistently creep back into our reflections" (p. 47). The only way to really see the world clearly is to remain as free as possible from preconceived ideas or notions, but van Manen asserts from Merleau-Ponty (1956) that complete reduction may never be possible because of the intimate relationship individuals have with the world. Merleau-Ponty (1956) further states that "The phenomenological world is not pure being, but the sense which is revealed where the paths of my various experiences intersect, and also where my own and other people intersect and engage each other like gears. It is thus inseparable from subjectivity and intersubjectivity which find their unity when I either take up my past experiences in those of the present, or other people's in my own" (p. xxii). During data collection and analysis, I made my orientation and pre-understanding of critical illness and critical care explicit and known, but held them deliberately at bay and bracketed them.

2.3.3.1.6 Afterthoughts Using phenomenology from Merleau-Ponty's philosophical perspective, this study shed light on the phenomenon of the ICU experience during critical illness from the perspectives of patients, family members, and nurses. Understanding the person's lived body and the notion that the experience of critical illness is dependent on the individual's embodied temporal, spatial, and relational horizons, rather than only naturalistic, biological, and physiological aspects, reveals a new conception of critical illness that will provide caregivers with knowledge about effective care. A better understanding and description of these experiences was revealed toward a more holistic, subjective consideration of a person's narrative and lifeworld, which opens new ways for coping among patients and their families, as well as new caregiving possibilities for nurses. The patient's experience as it relates to finding meaning during critical illness centers on obtaining support from their family and professionalism from their nurses. Adaptation in the ICU, as experienced by nurses, patients, and family members, integrates family as a unit, physical care/comfort, physiological care, and psychosocial support, resulting in transformation.

2.3.4 Descriptive or Hermeneutic/Interpretive Phenomenology?

Following in the footsteps of Husserl and Heidegger, many other philosophers have weighed in on the phenomenology problem, leading to even more confusion for the novice phenomenological researcher. First, phenomenology as a philosophy is classified based on the era of the phenomenologists writing on it, namely: early twentieth century phenomenology (Husserl, Heidegger, Scheler, and Stein); mid-twentieth century phenomenology (Patocka, Levinas, Sarte, Merleau-Ponty, de Beauvoir, Blanchot, Arendt, Gadamer, Marcel, Ricouer, Henry, and Derrida); and late twentieth and early twenty-first century phenomenology (Lingis, Ihde, Waldenfels, Serres, Nancy, Marion, Agamben, Stiegler, Figal, Romano, and Gosetti- Ferencei) (van Manen 2014). Second, these phenomenologists' philosophical perspectives are either purely descriptive (Edmund Husserl, Amedeo Giorgi, Paul Collaizi, Adrian van Kaam, Karin Dahlberg), hermeneutic/interpretive (Martin Heidegger, Hans George-Gadamer, Jean Luc Nancy, Max van Manen, Jonathan Smith, Karin Dahlberg, Patricia Benner), descriptive-hermeneutic (Maurice Merleau-Ponty, Max van Manen), or, more recently, hermeneutic reflective life-world research (Karin Dahlberg). These phenomenologists offer varied methodological and philosophical insights that may guide inquiries. It is not easy to place them in precise philosophical and historical frameworks. Each tradition helps researchers look at the world and at life in new and different ways (Smith and Liehr 1999). Across all of these perspectives, however, the philosophical assumptions rest on some common grounds: the lived experiences of persons, the view that these experiences are conscious ones, and the development of descriptions of the essences of these experiences, not explanations or analysis. The subjective character of experience and the importance of appreciating subjective experience when understanding other people are emphasized (Risjord 2010). Streubert and Carpenter (1999) state: "Making explicit the school of thought that guides an inquiry will help researchers conduct a credible study and help these people who use the findings apply the results within an appropriate context" (p. 19).

A discussion of all the phenomenological methodologies mentioned here is beyond the scope of this chapter, but exemplars applying Amedeo Giorgi's and Max van Manen's descriptive-hermeneutic approaches will be presented later, to add to the one already discussed using Merleau-Ponty's (1945/1962) phenomenological philosophy. Including these three exemplars will help new nurse researchers of phenomenology "picture" a full study from descriptive, hermeneutic/interpretive, and existential-embodied perspectives. Phenomenological studies conducted by nurse researchers are mostly underpinned by approaches based on Husserl and Heidegger, but more and more are using Merleau-Ponty's existential-embodied stance.

2.4 Phenomenology-as-Qualitative Research

Phenomenology is both a philosophy and a method (Eddles-Hirsch 2015; Merleau-Ponty 1945/1962). It is as much a way of thinking or perceiving as it is a method. Phenomenology as a method aims at researching rigorous knowledge and presupposes the existence of phenomena (Tarozzi and Mortari 2010). What is the phenomenological method? Phenomenological methodology cannot be reduced to a general set of strategies or research techniques (van Manen 2014). From Heidegger (1982), van Manen (2014) says: "It is difficult to describe phenomenological research methods since even within the tradition of philosophy itself, there is no such thing as one phenomenology, and if there could be such a thing it would never become anything like philosophical technique" (p. 41). There should be openness and acceptance with respect to the realization that phenomenology is a method consisting of methods (van Manen 2014). If Giorgi presents a "scientific phenomenology," van Manen rejects the idea of phenomenological method altogether (Paley 2017). He articulates that in his approach to a phenomenon, it is an interplay of six "activities." "Method" refers to the way or attitude of approaching a phenomenon. How we study phenomena influences what we find (Ironside 2005). How is nursing research that uses phenomenological methodologies perceived, now and in the past? Nursing research utilizing phenomenology as the guiding philosophy and as a method has always been questioned and criticized, going back decades.

Nursing studies have drawn on the philosophical tradition of phenomenology when conducting their qualitative inquiries, developing their own methodologies and theoretical foundations. This use and application of phenomenology has, however, not been met with universal approval (Zahavi and Martiny 2010). One prominent and persistent opponent has been John Paley. According to Zahavi and Martiny (2010), Paley (2017) has accused nurses of mostly misinterpreting the philosophical ideas, and has said that they should abandon their attempts to ground their research on phenomenological philosophy altogether. Aside from Paley (2017), Giorgi (2000a), Crotty (1996), Porter (2008), and Thomas (2005) all posit that nurse researchers using the phenomenological approach do not have a strong knowledge base or philosophical foundation to conduct this naturalistic study. A detailed discussion of this ongoing debate is beyond the scope of this chapter. The focus is rather on phenomenology as a method that is used in nursing research.

Scholars agree that phenomenology is an approach to human research (Dowling 2007; Earle 2010; Munhall 1994; van Manen 1990; Zahavi and Martiny 2010). Some nursing scholars noted for grounding their research and theory in phenomenology are: Patricia Benner, Rosemarie Rizzo Parse, Josephine Paterson and Lorraine Zderad, and Jean Watson. The discipline of nursing views phenomenology as an alternative to empirical science that offers a discerning means of understanding nursing phenomena specifically in relation to lived experience (Earle 2010; Giorgi 2000b; Norlyk and Harder 2010; Rapport and Wainwright 2006; Salmon 2012). Phenomenology is also consistent with the values of nursing practice, specifically the holistic view of a person, the meaning of their experiences, and the use of the self as a therapeutic tool (Earle 2010; Koch 1995; McConnell-Henry et al. 2009). Edward (2006) states:

Phenomenological methodology utilizes the patient's own language to reflect meanings embedded in their own experience. It is a process that accepts the validity of the person's descriptions and understandings, incorporates the perspective of the experience of the nurse, and produces an interpretative narrative of the experience. The patient's narratives have the potential to provide insight for the purpose of clinical process such as assessment and planning, providing a basis for identifying potential clinical interventions. Insight into the patient's lived world can engage the patient and/or his or her family members in a meaningful therapeutic alliance formed on the foundation of the essence of the person's lived experiences. (pp. 237–238)

Matua (2015), Biggerstaff and Thompson (2008), and Pringle et al. (2011) concur that phenomenology is attractive to nursing because it can help to improve care and understanding of issues critical to nurses and their clients, whether as individuals, families, or larger communities, through understanding of patients' unique experiences and how the patients interpret them. Thus, phenomenology is a well-substantiated qualitative methodology that is highly valuable for addressing research questions specific to the discipline of nursing. It is also essential for the implementation of holistic, empathic, and individualized nursing care (Earle 2010).

2.4.1 Amedeo Giorgi's Descriptive Phenomenology

Amedeo Giorgi, together with two other psychologists, van Kaam and Colazzi, belongs to the Duquesne School of Phenomenology. The three have all asserted their dissatisfaction with the limitations of empiricism, and argued that it is not the best philosophy for grounding the science of psychology, which should instead be based in the broader phenomenological theory of science. Giorgi (2006a) states: "Phenomenology is not against empiricism, but it is broader than empirical philosophy. That is because its method interrogates phenomena which are not reducible to facts" (p. 354). Giorgi pioneered the Duquesne Phenomenological Research Method (DPRM), but emphasized that this approach and its methods originated from Husserl (1983), as well as from Merleau-Ponty's (1945/1962) insights. He emphasized that the procedures for the descriptive research method were directed by phenomenological philosophical principles. The DPRM procedures he set forth are presented in Table 2.4.

Giorgi's (1985) phenomenological approach follows the Husserl (1983) tradition of decontextualization and recontextualization, using inductive reasoning to understand universals presented descriptively. Giorgi maintains that the object of phenomenological description is achieved "solely" through a direct grasping (intuiting) of the essential structure of phenomena as they show in consciousness. He also situates himself within the perspective of Merleau-Ponty's (1945/1962) descriptive-existential phenomenological method, applying reduction, search for essences, and a focus on the intentionality. The psychologist proposes a method that is theoretically grounded in phenomenological philosophy and yet treats empirically derived data.

Giorgi (1985, 2008) asserts that the search for the essential structure of a phenomenon entails that it should: (i) be descriptive, to avoid any kind of premature analysis or explanatory constructs; (ii) use imaginative variations, or the idea of taking the meaning of any experience exactly as it appears or is presented in consciousness and phenomenological human scientific reduction in order to achieve nomothetic, descriptive results (i.e., the invariant meaning-structure for the phenomenon); assuming the attitude of the phenomenological psychological reduction means that the researcher will *bracket* all knowledge that is not part of the given phenomenon (theories and past knowledge, as well as established beliefs that have come from the researcher's own past experience) and does not consider the phenomenon to exist precisely as it is being presented, or will withhold the positing of the existence of the given; (iii) search for essences (context-related; meaning structures are situated in specific situations); and (iv) make

Table 2.4 The Duquesne Phenomenological Research Method.

Ask a few participants from the lifeworld to describe an experience of the phenomenon that the researcher is interested in. No definition is given. What is sought is a description of a situation as lived and understood by the participant from the perspective of the natural attitude.

Researcher assumes the attitude of the phenomenological reduction, a psychological perspective, and a certain sensitivity toward the phenomenon being researched.

Researcher begins the process of discovering the psychologically relevant lived meanings in the data by reading the entire description to get a sense of the whole.

Researcher goes back to the beginning of the description and begins to reread the description in order to break it up into manageable parts called "meaning units."

Once the meaning units have been established, the researcher transforms the participant's natural attitude expressions into expressions that more adequately convey the psychological meanings contained in the natural attitude expressions with the help of imaginative variation.

Once all meaning units have been transformed, one uses the transformed meaning units as the basis for writing the typical structure of the experience.

Check structure against transformed meaning units in order to be sure that all key constituents are at least implicitly included. Once the structure is obtained, the researcher dialogues the structure with the transformed meaning units and raw data in order to elaborate in full the findings of the study. Dialogue with literature then follows.

Source: Giorgi, A. (2008). Concerning a serious misunderstanding of the essence of the phenomenological method in Psychology. *Journal of Phenomenological Psychology*, 39: 33–58.

use of intentionality (placed in human consciousness, the intentional act by which every human being is related to the world and objects). Giorgi's method has been used in many phenomenological studies of nurse researchers. His influence is also evident in nursing theory, such as in Watson's (1985) theory of caring and Parse's (2001) human becoming theory.

2.4.1.1 Formulating the Research Question

The initial phase of the process in phenomenological research begins with an acknowl-edgment that there is a need to understand a phenomenon from the point of view of lived experience in order to be able to discover its meaning (Englander 2012). The formulation of a research question in which the researcher delineates a focus of investigation is the first step. Giorgi (2008) asserts that the researcher certainly has some idea of what they are looking for but chooses not to define it in order to avoid any kind of premature analysis or explanatory constructs. Rather, the researcher *brackets* or puts aside their own understanding of the phenomenon. The qualitative phenomenological researcher seeks an ordinary person in the lifeworld and asks for a careful, concrete description of a situation in which the person has lived through the experience of the phenomenon being researched (Giorgi 2008). The aim is to discover the meaning of that particular phenomenon. One example of a research question using Giorgi's approach can be phrased in the following manner: "What is the lived persistent psychological meaning of early emotional memories?" (Englander 2012); alternatively, it could start like this: "What is the structure of the phenomenon. . .?" (Beck 2020).

2.4.1.2 Sampling

The selection of participants is the initial step in the data-gathering process. In Giorgi's (2009) approach, the phenomenological researcher is not primarily interested in knowing how many, or how often one has had a particular experience. Rather, Giorgi (1988) advocates that the inquirer understands what "representativeness" means for the phenomenological study, which will equate to other evaluative criteria such as validity and reliability. Further, the results of the study cannot be evaluated on the basis of a sampling method or the number of participants. The aim is to have a general knowledge and structure of the phenomenon. Thus, the number and the distribution are not known, but there is knowledge of whether the samples lived the experience that the investigator is looking for. To the common question, "How many interview subjects do I need?" Kvale (1994) answers: "Interview so many subjects that you find out what you need to know" (p. 165). Englander (2012) states: "On the other hand, if a researcher has a qualitative purpose and a qualitative research question, he or she seeks knowledge of the content of the experience, often in depth, to seek the meaning of a phenomenon, not 'how many' people who have experienced such phenomena" (p. 21). This means that the sample in descriptive phenomenology is small. Giorgi (2009) recommends at least three participants, because one or two would be too difficult for the researcher to handle in terms of their own imagination.

2.4.1.3 Data Collection

Giorgi (2009) emphasizes that the researcher collects data to gather the lived experience of a phenomenon from the participants through a traditional face-to-face interview or a written (or recorded) account of the experience. The focus is as complete a description as possible of the experience that the participant has lived through. According to Englander (2012), there is no prescribed way of doing a good phenomenological interview, but he suggests that one have a preliminary meeting with the research participants prior to the actual interview in order to establish trust, review ethical considerations, and complete consent forms. Giorgi (2009) emphasizes that the interviewer has to keep the descriptive criterion in mind throughout the process.

Later, the recorded interviews will be transcribed into text by the researcher in order to attain a depth of understanding of the experience, and to help in the transition to the first step in data analysis.

2.4.1.4 Data Analysis

Before delving into full data analysis, the researcher should first read and re-read the whole interview texts or protocols in order to get a sense of their overall meaning. The only goal here is to understand the language of the describer, in order to grasp a *sense of the whole* of the co-researcher's experience. No analysis should take place during this stage. Giorgi (1985) emphasizes that the general sense grasped after the reading of an entire text should not be interrogated or made explicit in any way. Primarily, it serves as a ground for the next step.

The next step is to divide the protocol into smaller *meaning units,* with the aim of discriminating between different units that express a self-contained meaning. Giorgi (2006b) advocates that for each of these meaning units, one should seek to discover, articulate, and explicate its psychological value and significance. He also asserts that the constant effort to clarify the meaning units leads the researcher to self-correction.

The units are next transformed into meanings that are expressed in psychological and phenomenological concepts. By using imaginative variation, the researcher begins to both follow the concrete experience and reflect about the different possibilities of the meanings of experiences. The aim is to arrive at the general category by going through the concrete expressions, and not by abstraction or formalization, which are selective according to the criteria accepted (Giorgi 1985).

In a final step, when the whole text or description is divided into meaning units, the researcher can analyze each of them easily. A final and single general analysis is done, in which the transformed meaning units from all the protocols of the study are integrated and synthesized in order to describe what all the descriptions have in common. Synthesis of the different findings is done in order to capture the essence of the experience under investigation and make a final consistent description of the psychological structure under study (Giorgi 1985). These transformations are combined to create a general description of the experience. Giorgi's method of analysis aims to uncover the meaning of a phenomenon as experienced through the identification of essential themes. Writing up the general structure then ensues. This is a clear-cut process that gives a structure to the analyses and justifies the decisions made while analyzing the data.

2.4.1.5 Exemplar: Applying Giorgi's Descriptive Phenomenology

Alexander et al. (2015) conducted a phenomenological descriptive study to describe and understand how "seasoned" psychiatric nurses in the mid-Atlantic region of the United States came to choose and remain in the specialty using Giorgi's phenomenological descriptive method. The sample included four male and four female participants between the ages of 28 and 60 years. Semi-structured audio-taped interviews were conducted, beginning with a broad opening: "Tell me how you chose a career in psychiatric nursing." Participants were also asked to reflect upon factors in their nursing education program that influenced a psychiatric mental health nursing (**PMHN**) career choice, as well as on why they remained in their specific specialty. The researchers employed Giorgi's methods for data analysis, which are: first read the entire transcription to get a sense of the whole, identifying meaning units in the narrative, coding units of meaning, comparing, and contrasting data to identify themes, and integrating themes into a coherent description of the phenomenon. Table 2.5 provides the sample three-step data analysis methodology that Alexander et al. (2015) used.

Findings showed three themes related to career choice: interest developed prior to or while in nursing school, personal relevance, and validation of potential. Three themes emerged related to retention: overcoming stereotypes to develop career pride,

Table 2.5 Sample of Giorgi's three-step data analysis and corresponding themes.

Examples of Significant Statements from Participants	Meaning Units Formulated Meanings Assigned to Statements	Common Experiences (Codes)	Transformation (Themes)
P2: "We became very good friends . . . she's more of a sister than my sister. She went down the wrong path . . . terrible relationships . . . addicted to heroin . . . and I just could not detach myself from trying to get her on the right path . . . and she's doing great now."	Successfully intervened with friends with mental illness	Personal experience: friend (with mental illness prior to entering PMHN)	Personal relevance
P3: "I was brought to the psych field because my childhood wasn't all that great and I knew there were some mistakes that were made, um, and I was actually, um received psychiatric treatment as a child and I knew it needed to be different . . . So, everything that I do for the children is what I wanted somebody to do for me – and they were not there to do that – and I want to be there."	Passionate desire to make a difference in others' treatment; desire to right wrongs	Personal experience: treatment (for mental illness prior to entering PMHN)	Personal relevance
P5: "My mom and my three aunts are all psych nurses. [Mom stated] . . . if you notice, nurses in high positions . . . most of them have a psych background. They have a skill set that enables them to move through the ranks?"	Comfort level with people with mental illness		Participants believed that their prior experiences had a direct bearing on their decision to enter PMHN
P6: "I have a history of mental illness in my family. I have a comfort level with chaos . . . having a clinical setting in which I can kind of bring that around and manage the milieu and bring a little order and calm to it, I think probably, is me working out some issues from childhood."	Working out family-of-origin issues	Personal experience: mental illness in family of origin	Participants connected their personal experiences to their passionate desire to enter PMHN to make a difference in clinical care for those with mental illness

Source: Alexander et al. (2015). Career choice and longevity in US psychiatric mental health nurses. *Issues in Mental Health Nursing, 36*(6): 447–454.

positive team dynamics, and remaining hopeful. These results have impact for nursing related to both recruitment and retention of psychiatric mental health registered nurses. Psychiatric nursing faculty play a critical role in solidifying interest in PMHN (recruitment). Nursing administrators and staff development personnel are instruments in retaining the psychiatric mental health nurses by providing educational offerings and helping them overcome the challenges to keep staff curious about, motivated for, and interested in PMHN.

2.4.2 Max van Manen's Descriptive-Hermeneutic Phenomenology

Max van Manen is an internationally known Dutch-born Canadian scholar from the Utrecht School of Phenomenology in the Netherlands. Van Manen (1990) has been involved in ongoing inquiries in phenomenology, pedagogy, and phenomenology of practice in professional contexts such as psychology, education, healthcare, public health, nursing, and social work, including a contemporary popularity among not only nurses but medical practitioners as well (Dowling 2007; Mak et al. 2003). His approach has been used by scholars and researchers worldwide. Van Manen's (1990, 2014) works are focused on the phenomenological research method, the meaning of the pedagogical relation, pedagogical tact, the pedagogy of self-identity in interpersonal relations, the pedagogy of recognition, and the meaning of writing in qualitative research.

Phenomenology tries to distinguish what is unique and what is the nature or essence of a phenomenon in order to better understand what a particular experience is like (van Manen 2001). In his book *Researching Lived Experience*, van Manen (1990) introduces and explicates a hermeneutic phenomenological approach to human science research and writing. However, other scholars describe van Manen's approach to phenomenology as both descriptive and hermeneutic/interpretive (Cohen and Omery 1994; Dowling 2007; Mortari and Sita in Paley 2017; Tarozzi and Mortari 2010). He combines the German tradition of "human science pedagogy" (hermeneutic/interpretive) with the Dutch movement of "phenomenological pedagogy" (more descriptive). "Human science" is used interchangeably with "phenomenology" and "hermeneutics" in his early works.

Van Manen (1990) asserts that hermeneutic phenomenological research is: (i) the study of lived experience; (ii) the explication of phenomena as they present themselves to consciousness; (iii) the study of essences; (iv) the description of the experiential meanings we live as we live them; (v) the human scientific study of phenomena (the attentive practice of thoughtfulness); (vi) the search for what it means to be human; and (vii) a poetizing activity. He emphasizes that to do hermeneutic phenomenology is to attempt to accomplish the impossible: to construct a full interpretive description of some aspect of the *lifeworld*. According to van Manen (1990), the lifeworld – the world of lived experience – is both the source and the object of phenomenological research. The basic things about the lifeworld are the experiences of lived body, lived space, lived time, and lived human relation (the four existentials). Van Manen also emphasizes that a real understanding of phenomenology can only be accomplished by "doing it."

The methodology of phenomenology posits an approach that has no pre-determined set of fixed procedures, techniques, and concepts that would rule the research study.

In other words, phenomenology and hermeneutics has no method (van Manen 1990, p. 30)! Rather, hermeneutical phenomenological research may be seen as a dynamic interplay among six research activities: (i) turning to the phenomenon that seriously interests us and commits us to the world; (ii) investigating experience as we live it rather than as we conceptualize it; (iii) reflecting on the essential themes that characterize the phenomenon; (iv) describing the phenomenon through the art of writing and rewriting; (v) maintaining a strong and oriented pedagogical relation to the phenomenon; and (vi) balancing the research context by considering parts and whole.

2.4.2.1 Formulating a Phenomenological Research Question

After identifying the specific interest from a selected human experience (phenomenon), a research question is posed. To question phenomenologically is to ask, "What is something really like?" or, "What is the nature of experience?" The phenomenological question must not only be made clear and understood by the researcher, but must also be "lived" by them (van Manen 1990).

2.4.2.2 Data Collection

Data collection, according to van Manen (1990), is the gathering of other people's experiences or experiential materials with an emphasis always on the meaning of those lived experiences. A conversational interview is one method of gathering data, be they in the form of stories, life stories, anecdotes, or recollections of experiences. Van Manen emphasizes that as we interview others about their experiences of a certain phenomenon, it is important to stay close to the experience as lived, and to be very concrete. It is also not necessary to ask many questions, but rather the person should be allowed to gather their recollections and proceed with their story. Interviews can at times be an occasion to reflect with the interviewee or with collaborators in the research study. This is called hermeneutic interviewing.

Close observation is another method of collecting experiential descriptions. According to van Manen (1990), close observation involves entering the lifeworld of the persons whose experiences are relevant study material for the research. He cautions naturalistic investigators against too simplistic interpretations and against having a manipulative and artificial attitude when observing a participant. He states: "The best way to enter a person's lifeworld is to participate in it" (p. 69). A careful reflectivity and hermeneutic alertness are also essential for close observation. There are other ways of collecting experiential material: literature, poetry, biographies, autobiographies, diaries, journals and logs, and art (e.g., painting, sculpture, music, and cinematography) (van Manen 1990).

2.4.2.3 Data Analysis

Van Manen (1990) emphasizes that the structure and meaning of the lived experience (lived through as *wholes*) have to be made explicit. This involves a process of reflectively appropriating and clarifying in order to have an insight into the essence of the phenomenon from the experience. Reflecting on experience then becomes a matter of analyzing the structural and thematic aspects of the experience. Thematic analysis is done to illuminate phenomenological themes, which are the experiential structures of the experience that are embodied. Themes are not objects or generalizations. There are three approaches to uncovering the thematic aspects of a phenomenon: (i) the wholistic or sententious approach, which involves attending to the text as a whole; (ii) the selective or highlighting approach, which involves looking for and underlining or highlighting texts or phrases that seem particularly essential or revealing about the phenomenon; and (iii) the detailed or line-by-line approach, which involves closely examining every single sentence, or sentences (van Manen 1990).

Once the themes are illuminated, van Manen (1990) emphasizes that the researcher can go back to the participants and engage in a hermeneutic conversation. This is done so participants can reflect on their experiences and further determine the meanings of these experiences. This is a sort of collaboration between the researcher and the participant that results in interpretive conversation. Collaborative interpretive conversation may also be done by a research group or seminar. Van Manen (1990) articulates that lived experience – its structures and meanings – can also be described and interpreted using the four "existentials" of the lifeworld.

These four fundamental existentials of corporeality, spatiality, temporality, and relationality are based on Merleau-Ponty's (1945/1962) existential-embodied philosophy. Corporeality (lived body) refers to the fact that people are always *bodily* in the world. Spatiality is *lived space*. A lived body occupies a lived space. Temporality is *lived time* – a person's temporal way of being in the world. Relationality is *lived relation*. Persons maintain a lived relation with others, and also share an interpersonal space with them. A detailed discussion of the four existentials is provided in Section 2.3.3. After completing data analysis and illuminating the themes, the researcher has to embark on hermeneutic phenomenological writing.

Human science research is a form of writing. Van Manen (1990) states that "This means that in phenomenological human science, the process of writing involves more than merely communicating information." He asserts that interpretive phenomenological research and theorizing cannot be separated from the textual practice of writing. The textual quality or form of our writing also cannot be separated from the content or text. Writing is a reflexive activity that creates signifying relations, a pattern of meaningful relation condensed into a discursive whole (theory), and it mediates action. Writing is not just the last step of the phenomenological research process. To write is to measure our thoughtfulness, and it exercises our ability to see (van Manen 1990).

2.4.2.4 On Saturation

Van Manen (2002/2016) posits that data saturation is *inappropriate* in phenomenology, and that there is no saturation point with respect to phenomenological meaning. Some would disagree, but he emphasizes that one cannot catch all the meaning or meaningfulness of a human phenomenon. Every phenomenological topic can be explored over and over for dimensions of originary meaning and aspects of meaningfulness (van Manen 2002/2016). In other words, researchers cannot say that they have uncovered all the meaning of a phenomenon at hand (Beck 2020). Thus, van Manen (1990) does not prescribe a typical sample size.

2.4.2.5 Exemplar: Applying van Manen's Approach to the Lived Critical Care Experiences of Patients, Family Members, and Nurses in the Emergency Department

The phenomenon of interest for this qualitative phenomenological study was the experience of nurses, patients, and family members in the emergency department (**ED**). The aim was to explore, understand, and describe their lived experiences of during critical illness in the ED. Understanding the experiences of nurses, patients, and family members is important in determining the factors that shape these experiences and other aspects of emergency care. The ultimate goal was to contribute knowledge that would potentially impact the provision of emergency care and improvement of patient outcomes. The following research questions guided this study: (i) What are the patients' and their families' experiences of the nurse in an ED environment? (ii) What are the nurses' experiences of the patients and family members in an ED environment? (Cypress 2013, 2014).

2.4.2.5.1 Research Design In this study, the descriptive-hermeneutic phenomenological method as described by van Manen (1990) was used. Van Manen explicitly connects phenomenological and hermeneutical approaches in human research (Mortari and Sita in Tarozzi and Mortari 2010). His approach is usually labeled as hermeneutic, but other scholars perceive that it is a combination of both descriptive and hermeneutic approaches. Mortari and Sita (Tarozzi and Mortari 2010) state that "In van Manen's perspective, phenomenological knowledge is both descriptive and interpretive, interpretive, since it mediates between interpreted meanings and the thing toward which interpretation point" (pp. 137–138). Phenomenology uses an inductive approach, and is a pure description of the lifeworld – the world as immediately experienced, rather than as conceptualized (van Manen 1990). Phenomenological description lies in interpretation via some "text" or symbolic form, or is hermeneutic. Van Manen's hermeneutic phenomenological method helped explicate the phenomenon of the lived experiences of nurses, patients, and family members during critical illness in the ED. He asserts that a hermeneutic phenomenological research is a dynamic interplay among six research activities: (i) turning to the phenomenon that seriously interests us and commits us to the world; (ii) investigating experience as we live it rather than as we conceptualize it; (iii) reflecting on the essential themes that characterize the phenomenon; (iv) describing the phenomenon through the art of writing and rewriting; (v) maintaining a strong and oriented pedagogical relation to the phenomenon; and (vi) balancing the research context by considering parts, and whole (van Manen 1990).

2.4.2.5.2 Setting and Sample The study was approved by the university and hospital institutional review boards (**IRBs**). A purposive method of sampling was used to recruit participants on the basis of their knowledge and experience of critical illness in the ED. The 10 patient participants in this study were acutely, critically ill patients in the ED prior to their transfer to either the regular medical floor or the ICU. Patient participants included six men and four women ranging in age from 39 to 53 years. The sample of five family members included patients' spouses, a daughter, a son, and a patient's mother, all of whom were with the patients in the ED. These family members were the patients' immediate family, primary support system, or caregivers. The family members included two men and three women, ranging in age from 28 to 66 years (Cypress 2013, 2014).

2.4.2.5.3 Data Collection and Analysis The data were collected over six months (500 hours in the research setting; 50-plus hours of taped interviews) during the year 2010. Data collection for the nurse, patient, and family member participants consisted of two 45-minute to one-hour audiotaped interviews, which took place in a private room on the medical floors where the patients were transferred. The interviews were conducted after the patients had been discharged from the ED, and while they were fully awake and alert in the medical-surgical floors. Nurses were interviewed in a private place convenient for them. The interview style was based on van Manen's (1990) unstructured or open-ended interview. It was used as a means for exploring and gathering narratives (or stories) of lived experiences, allowing participants the freedom to respond to questions and probes and to narrate their experiences without being tied down to specific answers (Ajjawi and Higgs 2007). A common thread noted, aside from patients' perceptions of their lived experiences, was the behaviors expected of an ED nurse (Cypress 2013, 2014).

At the end of every interview, the participants were given the opportunity to review and modify the data. As the sole instrument of the study, the researcher worked closely together with the participants to collect the data. The researcher's role in this study was as a participant observer, interviewer, and analyzer of data. Data analysis was accomplished using van Manen's (1990) wholistic, selective, and detailed line-by-line approach. Van Manen (1990) states that "Any lived experience is an appropriate source for uncovering thematic aspects of the phenomenon it describes" (p. 92). Themes and descriptors were illuminated and interpreted to achieve an understanding of the perceived phenomenon as experienced by the participants in this study. Methodological rigor was achieved using the criteria of credibility, transferability, dependability, and confirmability (Guba and Lincoln 1994). A detailed discussion of rigor is given in Chapter 3.

2.4.2.5.4 Findings Five essential themes and corresponding descriptors emerged from the thematic analysis of the participants' narratives. The three themes from the patients and their families were critical thinking, communication, and sensitivity and caring. The two themes that the nurses illuminated were their response to physiological deficits and their view of patients and families as co-participants in the human care processes. These themes constituted the perceived experiences of the nurses and of patients and their families in the ED (Cypress 2013, 2014).

2.4.2.5.5 Afterthoughts The findings of this qualitative phenomenological study indicate that patients' and family members' perceptions of nurses in the ED relate to their critical thinking skills, communication, sensitivity, and caring abilities. Nurses identified that response to patients' physiological deficits was paramount in the ED, and that involving the patients and families in the human care processes would help in this respect. Emergency nurses and staff may embrace family presence, and this leads to benefits for family members when the practice is well established. This study supports recognizing the patient and family as active participants and key decision-makers in the patient's medical care; encouraging family member presence; and creating institutional policies for patient–family-centered care. The organization plays a key role in encouraging family-centered care by providing appropriate education and support to nursing staff. Mentoring, leading, facilitating, providing stress management, and promoting the psychological and emotional well-being of nurses are also encouraged in order to improve job satisfaction and performance and thus contribute to better patient–family satisfaction and outcomes.

2.4.3 Conceptual versus Theoretical Framework

Apart from knowing the philosophical assumptions, paradigms, and underpinnings of a qualitative research study, the researcher has to be aware that qualitative research is not conducted just to answer research questions, but also to develop theories. This is one confusion that arise among novice naturalistic investigators and students (Collins and Stockton 2018; Cypress 2015; Merriam and Tisdell 2016). The terms "conceptual" and "theoretical" framework create a perplexity among researchers (Collins and Stockton 2018) and are used interchangeably in the literature (Merriam and Tisdell 2016). This equivocation may happen because established researchers have varying perspectives on how conceptual and theoretical components function (Collins and Stockton 2018). Scholars and investigators like Maxwell (2005) and Merriam and Tisdell (2016) prefer the term "theoretical framework" to "conceptual" because they use the terms in a broader sense. Thus, "theoretical framework" includes terms, concepts, models, thoughts, and ideas, as well as references to specific theories (Collins and Stockton 2018). Additionally, some qualitative inquirers like Maxwell (2005) state that the two terms are "almost" the same.

Aside from all this perplexity and incongruency, the bigger continuing debate is whether to use a theoretical framework in a qualitative study. This perspective and its details are beyond the scope of this chapter. Nevertheless, it is beneficial to mention that there are a number of proponents of the use of theory in a naturalistic inquiry. Collins and Stockton (2018) mention researchers like Ravitch and Carl (2016), Merriam and Tisdell (2016), Anfara and Mertz (2015), and Saldana (2015) in this regard.

Questions commonly asked by novice researchers include: "Do I use a conceptual or a theoretical framework?" "Should I use a framework from the beginning, or later, or not at all?" "When should I introduce a framework?" An expert qualitative adviser should be able to guide the novice embarking on a phenomenological research journey. Table 2.6 explains the differences between conceptual and theoretical frameworks.

A theory is an organized and systematic set of interrelated statements that specify the nature of relationships between two or more variables with the purpose of understanding a problem or the nature of things (Streubert and Carpenter 1999). Theories provide the structure of a research study, and are used to inform its ontological, methodological, and evaluative commitments. Quantitative researchers collect facts through empirical investigations in order to explain and predict phenomena using a pre-existing theory from the beginning of a study in order to guide it, reflecting a deductive theory-testing approach. Specific hypotheses can be deduced from a theory, which serves as a more general statement of interrelated phenomena that helps unveil existing relationships. This is referred to as the *theoretical framework* of a study. It is the application of concepts

Table 2.6 Conceptual versus theoretical framework.

Element	Conceptual Framework	Theoretical Framework
Inception	Evolves from the researcher's synthesis of empirical and theoretical findings from the literature	Stems from pre-existing theory and logical review of literature
Purpose	Clarifies concepts and proposes relationships among concepts in identified phenomenon; provides context for interpreting the study findings	Explains the relationship between two or more variables; provides and guides the researcher with the overall methodology (research design, sampling, data collection, analysis and interpretation; standardized context or none)
Review of Literature Process	Mainly inductive, oriented toward discovery or theory-developing approach	Reflects a deductive approach; hypothesis is deduced from a theory to unveil existing relationships; utilizes a theory-testing approach
Methodological Approach	Qualitative research in general but may be used in quantitative and mixed-methods research; data are collected from interviews, observations, descriptive surveys but may include empirical surveys	Mainly quantitative research; data are collected from empirical and experimental investigations (surveys and tests)
Application	Less formal structure and limited to specific problem and context	More formal and wider application beyond the identified problem and context

Source: Based on Imenda, S. (2014). Is there a conceptual difference between theoretical and conceptual frameworks? *Journal of Social Science*, 38(2): 185–195.

of a theory to offer an explanation or shed some light on a particular phenomenon or research problem.

Discussions of theory in qualitative research relate to the theories that ground a methodological approach (phenomenology, ethnography, narrative research) or to the epistemological paradigms that guide a study (postpositivist, constructivist, critical) (Collins and Stockton 2018). Qualitative research is supposed to begin *without* a prior theory. The essence of qualitative studies, after all, is *theory-building* using an inductive approach. A phenomenon in qualitative research cannot meaningfully be studied in reference to only one theory. The researcher may have to synthesize both empirical and theoretical findings from the literature in order to ascertain the current knowledge on a problem or phenomenon. This synthesis may be called the *conceptual framework*.

A conceptual framework is an end result of bringing together a number of related concepts to describe and give a broader and more holistic understanding of the phenomenon of interest. In other words, a conceptual framework is loosely defined as a map of how all of the literature works together in a particular study (Collins and Stockton 2018). A conceptual framework is something that is *constructed*, not found or "ready-made." The process of arriving at a conceptual framework is an inductive one oriented toward discovery or theory-developing (Smith and Liehr 1999). Qualitative research is based on a constructivist epistemology, and explores what it assumes to be a socially constructed dynamic reality through a framework that is value-laden, flexible, descriptive, holistic, and context-sensitive (Guba and Lincoln 1994).

Findings illuminated through qualitative research may lead to the development of yet unknown theories. Maxwell (2005) asserts that qualitative studies utilizing any methodological choice may result in theory construction. Grounded theory explicitly calls for the construction of a theory from a study's findings during the research process. While generally phenomenology tries to push off theory in the sense of abstractive science, it may also bring in theory when exploring a human phenomenon or event (van Manen 2014). Concepts and constructs represented in qualitative research methodologies represent a form of theory, and are theory-driven. Thus, it is generally accepted that qualitative research findings have the potential to create a theory (Streubert and Carpenter 1999).

In summary, both "conceptual" and "theoretical" frameworks refer to the *epistemological paradigm* a qualitative researcher adopts in viewing the phenomenon of interest. Both frameworks let the investigator understand the rationale and assumptions underlying the study of a particular topic, give an appropriate structure for the inquiry, conceptually ground the study approach, and provide meaningful interpretation of results. There is also the matter of the use of interpretive frameworks or theoretical lenses in qualitative inquiries. We have discussed how, ideally, a qualitative study should not commence using a theory that creates confusion among researchers. Interpretive positions, if used, provide a perspective on all aspects of a qualitative study (Scotland 2012). The aim of these theories is social justice, where the study ends with distinct steps toward reform and a call for action. Interpretive communities in this regard include the postmodern perspective, feminist theories, critical theories, queer theories, and disability theories. A description of these frameworks is beyond the scope of this chapter. Table 2.6 presents the differences between the conceptual and theoretical frameworks as they relate to a study's inception, purpose, literature review, methodological approach, and application (Imenda 2014).

2.5 Conclusion

Qualitative research, and the larger discussion about the philosophical, paradigmatic, conceptual, and interpretive frameworks that researchers bring to a study, is complex and not without disagreements. Phenomenology as a research approach provides an avenue for investigation that allows for a description of the lived experiences of phenomena that are important in nursing practice. This chapter discussed the phenomenological philosophies of Husserl, Heidegger, and Merleau-Ponty, as well as Giorgi's and van Manen's approaches. It also presented exemplars from actual descriptive, hermeneutic/interpretive, and existential-embodied phenomenological research studies.

References

Ajjawi, R. and Higgs, J. (2007). Using hermeneutic phenomenology to investigate how experienced practitioners learn to communicate clinical reasoning. *The Qualitative Report* 12 (4): 612–638.

Alexander, R.K., Diefenbeck, C.A., Carlton, G., and Brown, C.G. (2015). Career choice and longevity in US psychiatric mental health nurses. *Issues in Mental Health Nursing* 36 (6): 447–454.

Anfara, V.A. and Mertz, N.T. (2015). *Theoretical Frameworks in Qualitative Research*, 2e. Sage Publications.

Beck, C. (2020). *Introduction to Phenomenology. Focus on Methodology*. Sage Publications.

Benner, P. and Wrubel, J. (1989). *The Primacy of Caring*. Addison-Wesley.

Biggerstaff, D. and Thompson, A.R. (2008). Interpretative phenomenological analysis (IPA): a qualitative methodology of choice in healthcare research. *Qualitative Research in Psychology* 5 (3): 214–224.

Cohen, M.Z. and Omery, A. (1994). Schools of phenomenology: implications for research. In: *Critical Issues in Qualitative Research Methods* (ed. J.M. Morse), 136–156. Sage Publications.

Collins, C.S. and Stockton, C.M. (2018). The central role of theory in qualitative research. *International Journal of Qualitative Methods* 17: 1–10.

Creswell, J.W. (2007). *Qualitative Inquiry and Research Design: Choosing among Five Approaches*. Sage Publications.

Crotty, M. (1996). *Phenomenology and Nursing Research*. Churchill Livingstone.

Cypress, B. (2013). Using the synergy model of patient care in understanding the lived emergency department experiences of patients, family members and their nurses during critical illness: a phenomenological study. *Dimensions of Critical Care Nursing* 32 (6): 310–321.

Cypress, B. (2014). The emergency room: experiences of patients, families, and their nurses. *Advanced Emergency Nursing* 36 (2): 164–176.

Cypress, B. (2015). Qualitative research: the "what," "why," "who," and "how"! *Dimensions of Critical Care Nursing* 34 (6): 356–361.

Dilthey, W. (1985). *Poetry and Experience. Selected Works*, vol. V. Princeton University Press.

Dowling, M. (2007). From Husserl to van Manen. A review of different phenomenological approaches. *International Journal of Nursing Studies* 44: 131–142.

Earle, V. (2010). Phenomenology as research method or substantive metaphysics?: an overview of phenomenology's uses in nursing. *Nursing Philosophy* 11 (4): 286–296.

Eddles-Hirsch, K. (2015). Phenomenology and educational research. *International Journal of Advanced Research* 3 (8): 251–260.

Edward, K.L. (2006). A theoretical discussion about the clinical value of phenomenology for nurses. *Holistic Nursing Practice* 20 (5): 235–238.

Englander, M. (2012). The interview: data collection in descriptive phenomenological human scientific research. *Journal of Phenomenological Psychology* 43: 13–35.

Evans, M.K. and O'Brien, B. (2005). Gestational diabetes: the meaning of an at-risk pregnancy. *Qualitative Health Research* 15 (1): 66–81.

Farrell, M.E., Joseph, D.H., and Schwartz-Barcott, D.S. (2005). Visiting hours in the ICU: finding the balance among patient, visitor and staff. *Nursing Forum* 20 (1): 18–28.

Giorgi, A. (1985). *Phenomenology and Psychological Research*. Duquesne University Press.

Giorgi, A. (1988). Validity and reliability from a phenomenological perspective. In: *Recent Trends in Theoretical Psychology* (eds. W.J. Baker, L.P. Mos, H.V. Rappard and H.J. Stam), 27–36. Springer.

Giorgi, A. (2000a). The status of Husserlian phenomenology in caring research. *Scandinavian Journal of Caring Science* 14: 3–10.

Giorgi, A. (2000b). Concerning the application of phenomenology to caring research. *Scandinavian Journal of Caring Science* 14: 11–15.

Giorgi, A. (2006a). Difficulties encountered in the application of the phenomenological method in the social sciences. *Análise Psicológica* (2006) 3 (XXIV): 353–361.

Giorgi, A. (2006b). Concerning variations in the application of the phenomenological method. *The Humanistic Psychologist* 34 (4): 305–319.

Giorgi, A. (2008). Concerning a serious misunderstanding of the essence of the phenomenological method in psychology. *Journal of Phenomenological Psychology* 39: 33–58.

Giorgi, A. (2009). *The Descriptive Phenomenological Method in Psychology: A Modified Husserlian Approach*. Duquesne University Press.

Guba, E.G. and Lincoln, Y.S. (1994). Competing paradigms in qualitative research. In: *Handbook of Qualitative Research* (eds. N.K. Denzin and Y.S. Lincoln), 105–117. Sage Publications.

Heidegger, M. (1927/1962). *Being and Time*. SCM Press.

Heidegger, M. (1982). *The Basic Problems of Phenomenology*. University Press.

Heidegger, M. (1992). *History of the Concept of Time* (trans. T. Kiesel). University Press.

Husserl, E. (1973). *Cartesian Meditations. An Introduction to Phenomenology* (trans. D. Cairns). Martinus Nijhoff Publisher.

Husserl, E. (1981). Phenomenology and anthropology. In: *Husserl Shorter Works* (eds. P. McCormick and F. Elliston), 315–323) (trans. R.G. Schmitt. University of Notre Dame.

Husserl, E. (1983). *Ideas Pertaining to Pure Phenomenology and to a Phenomenological Philosophy* (trans. D. Carr). First Book: Martinus Nijhoff Publisher (trans. F. Kersten). Northwestern University Press.

Imenda, S. (2014). Is there a conceptual difference between theoretical and conceptual frameworks? *Journal of Social Science* 38 (2): 185–195.

Ironside, P. (2005). *Beyond Method: Philosophical Conversations in Healthcare Research and Scholarship*. University of Wisconsin Press.

Kaufer, S. and Chemero, A. (2015). *Phenomenology an Introduction*. Polity Press.

Koch, T. (1995). Interpretive approaches in nursing research: the influence of Husserl and Heidegger. *Journal of Advanced Nursing* 21 (5): 827–836.

Kvale, S. (1994). Ten standard objections to qualitative research interviews. *Journal of Phenomenological Psychology* 25 (2): 147–173.

Lusardi, P., Jodka, P., Stambovsky, M. et al. (2011). The going home initiative: getting critical care patients home with hospice. *Critical Care Nurse* 31: 46–57.

Mak, Y.W., Elwyn, G., and Finlay, I.G. (2003). Patients' voices are needed in debates on euthanasia. *BMJ* 327 (7408): 213–215.

Matua, G.A. (2015). Choosing phenomenology as a guiding philosophy for nursing research. *Nurse Researcher* 22 (4): 50–34.

Maxwell, J.A. (2005). *Qualitative Research Design: An Interactive Approach*, 2e. Sage Publications.

McConnell-Henry, T., Chapman, Y., and Francis, K. (2009). Husserl and Heidegger: exploring the disparity. *International Journal of Nursing Practice* 15 (1): 7–15.

Merleau-Ponty, M. (1945/1962). *Phenomenology of Perception* (trans. C. Smith). Routledge & Kegan Paul.

Merleau-Ponty, M. (1956). What is phenomenology? *Cross Currents* 6: 59–70.

Merleau-Ponty, M. (1964). *The Primacy of Perception* (trans. J. Edie). Northwestern University Press.

Merriam, S.B. (2002). *Qualitative Research in Practice: Examples for Discussion and Analysis*, 1e. Jossey-Bass.

Merriam, S.B. and Tisdell, E.J. (2016). *Qualitative Research: A Guide to Design and Implementation*. Jossey-Bass.

Morse, J.M. (1991). *Qualitative Nursing Research: A Contemporary Dialogue*. Sage Publications.

Morse, J.M., Swanson, J.J., and Kuzel, A.J. (2001). *The Nature of Qualitative Evidence*. Sage Publications.

Moustakas, C. (1994). *Phenomenological Research Methods*. Sage Publications.

Munhall, P.L. (1994). *Revisioning Phenomenology: Nursing and Health Science Research*. National League of Nursing.

Norlyk, A. and Harder, I. (2010). What makes a phenomenological study phenomenological? An analysis of peer-reviewed empirical nursing studies. *Qualitative Health Research* 20 (3): 420–431.

Paley, J. (2017). *Phenomenology as Qualitative Research: A Critical Analysis of Meaning Attribution*. Routledge.

Parse, R.R. (2001). *Qualitative Inquiry: The Path of Sciencing*. Jones and Bartlett Publishers.

Porter, S. (2008). Nursing research and the cults of phenomenology. *Journal of Research in Nursing* 13 (4): 267–268.

Pringle, J., Drummond, J., McLafferty, E., and Hendry, C. (2011). Interpretative phenomenological analysis: a discussion and critique. *Nurse Researcher* 18 (3): 20–24.

Rapport, F. and Wainwright, P. (2006). Phenomenology as a paradigm of movement. *Nursing Inquiry* 13 (3): 228–236.

Ravitch, S.M. and Carl, N.M. (2016). *Qualitative Research: Bridging the Conceptual, Theoretical, and Methodological*. Sage.

Risjord, M. (2010). *Nursing Knowledge: Science, Practice and Philosophy*. Wiley.

Sadala, M. and Adorno, R. (2002). Phenomenology as a method to investigate the lived experience: a perspective from Husserl and Merleau-Ponty's thought. *Journal of Advanced Nursing* 37 (3): 282–293.

Saldana, J. (2015). *Thinking Qualitatively: Methods of Mind*. Sage Publications.

Salmon, J. (2012). The use of phenomenology in nursing research. *Nurse Researcher* 19 (3): 4–5.

Sandelowski, M. (2000). Focus on research methods whatever happened to qualitative description? *Research in Nursing & Health* 23: 334–340.

Scotland, J. (2012). Exploring the philosophical underpinnings of research: relating ontology and epistemology to the methodology and methods of the scientific, interpretive, and critical research paradigms. *English Language Teaching* 5 (9): 9–16.

Shem, S. (1978). *The House of God*. Dell Publishing.

Smith, M.J. and Liehr, P. (1999). Attentively embracing story: a middle-range theory with practice and research implications. *Research and Theory for Nursing Practice* 13 (3): 187–204.

Solomon, R.C. (1974). *Existentialism*. McGraw-Hill Humanities.

Streubert, H.J. and Carpenter, D.R. (1999). *Qualitative Research in Nursing: Advancing the Humanistic Imperative*, 3e. Lippincott Williams & Wilkins.

Tarozzi, M. and Mortari, L. (2010). *Phenomenology and Human Research Theory*. Zeta Books.

Thomas, S.P. (2005). Through the lens of Merleau-Ponty: advancing the phenomenological approach to nursing research. *Nursing Philosophy* 6: 63–76.

van Manen, M. (1990). *Researching Lived Experience: Human Science for an Action Sensitive Pedagogy*. State University Press.

van Manen, M. (2001). Professional practice and "doing phenomenology". In: *Handbook of Phenomenology and Medicine* (ed. S.K. Toombs), 457–474. Kluwer Press.

van Manen, M. (ed.) (2002/2016). *Writing in the Dark: Phenomenological Studies in Interpretive Inquiry*. Routledge.

van Manen, M. (2014). *Phenomenology of Practice: Meaning-Giving Methods in Phenomenological Research and Writing*. Left Coast Press.

Walsh, K. (1999). Shared humanity and the psychiatric nurse-patient encounter. *New Zealand Journal of Mental Health* 8: 2–8.

Watson, J. (1985). *Nursing: Human Science and Human Care: A Theory of Nursing*. Little Brown and Company.

Zahavi, D. and Martiny, K.M. (2010). Phenomenology in nursing studies: new perspectives. *International Journal of Nursing Studies* 93: 155–162.

Zussman, R. (1992). *Intensive Care: Medical Ethics and the Medical Profession*. Chicago University Press.

II

Methods of Phenomen-ological Data Collection, Reduction, Analysis, Inter-pretation, and Presentation

3

Collecting, Organizing, Analyzing, and Presenting Qualitative Data

Qualitative researchers set out clear goals and objectives at the beginning of a research study. A clear understanding of the aims motivating your work will help avoid you losing your way or spending time and effort doing things that don't advance your research (Maxwell 2005). These aims may often refer to collecting and analyzing data on a phenomenon that has been identified to be significant, relevant, and warranting exploration, description, and understanding. If your data collection and analysis are based on personal desires, without careful assessment of the implications of the latter for your methods and conclusions, you are in danger of creating a flawed or biased study (Maxwell 2005).

Data collection and analysis only begin after the preliminary steps of the research design have been fully implemented. Once we have identified a phenomenon that seriously interests us, and which commits us to the world, we may ask a research question that has the potential to help elucidate this phenomenon. The research question is the starting point, and the primary determinant of the study design. The naturalistic inquirer then determines what settings or individuals to select (using purposeful sampling), observe, or interview and what other sources of information to use. Consequently, they plan how to gather the information (data collection) and what to do with it in order to make sense of it (data analysis). The qualitative inquirer is the sole instrument of the study, and the research relationships are the means by which the research gets done (Maxwell 2005).

One vital issue in designing a qualitative study is to what extent one should decide on the methods in advance, rather than developing and modifying them during the process. Qualitative research is inductively grounded and based on philosophical and ethical grounds (Maxwell 2005). There is always the question whether to use structured or unstructured approaches in collecting the data. Structured approaches are identified with quantitative research that can help to ensure comparability of data across individuals, times, settings, and researchers. Unstructured approaches allow a focus on the particular phenomenon being studied, which may differ from others and requires individually tailored methods (Maxwell 2005). The strategy of triangulation is another aspect to consider in order to reduce the risks that study conclusions will reflect only systematic biases or limitations of a specific method. Triangulation affords

Fundamentals of Qualitative Phenomenological Nursing Research, First Edition. Brigitte S. Cypress.
© 2022 John Wiley & Sons Ltd. Published 2022 by John Wiley & Sons Ltd.

a broader understanding of the phenomenon under investigation. The data collection strategies will also go through a period of focusing and revision even if the study is carefully designed. This is because design in qualitative inquiries is emergent, enabling the researcher to better provide the data that will address the research questions and the plausible validity threats to the answers.

A qualitative researcher should be versatile enough to view a setting and recognize the restrictions in the types of data that can be collected (Denzin and Lincoln 1998). A "good" investigator is not confined methodologically by being trained in and limited to a single strategy. Such restrictions limit the results that can be obtained, and the strength of the study. Denzin and Lincoln (1998) state: "Productive data collection is the most exciting phase of qualitative inquiry" (p. 74). Time, effort, determination, persistence, and perseverance are essential for order and understanding to emerge, such that the patterns of relationships are illuminated, theoretical insights and linkages between categories are increased, and themes emerge. The processes of sampling, data collection, and analysis are concurrent, and continue until saturation is achieved. The use of data management methods is also important for the efficiency of the study. This includes transcription of audio-recorded interviews and the use of various qualitative data analysis software (**QDAS**) tools.

Data collection, management, and analysis are essential to qualitative research studies. When implemented properly, these processes enhance the quality and rigor of naturalistic inquiries. However, early-career researchers and doctoral students face challenges with these vital research steps, and they are often neglected aspects of qualitative research (Devers and Frankel 2014).

3.1 Ethical Considerations

Data collection involves more than the different forms of data and the procedures for collecting them. It involves consideration of the ethical issues involved in gaining entry to and approval from the research site, protection of the rights of the participants including informed consents, choosing and conducting an appropriate sampling strategy, planning the mode of recording information, storing the data securely, and proper use and dissemination of findings (Creswell and Poth 2017). Interviews should be fully overt (Lincoln and Guba 1991). Whether structured or unstructured, respondents should be fully and completely informed that an interview is taking place, and how many times, for what purpose, and in what way the resulting information will be used. Interviews entail certain steps, and are at times conducted more than once. The researcher should prepare for the interview, take initial steps, pace the interview according to how the interviewees respond, and keep the process productive. Respondents should also be prepared by the researcher for the termination of the interview, and thus gain closure from the interactions. Courtesy demands that the interviewer thanks the respondents for their cooperation (Lincoln and Guba 1991). Similarly, in observation as a method for collecting data, permission should be obtained to gain access to the research site, participants should sign the informed consent, the type of observation should be determined, and care should be undertaken in recording and storing data to protect the privacy and confidentiality of the information. Observations should also be overt.

3.2 Data Collection Strategies

Data collection is a series of interrelated activities aimed at gathering information to answer emerging research questions (Creswell 2007). The initial design of a qualitative inquiry should have provision for the kinds of data collection activities that will likely be done at different stages of the study. Data can be collected from more than one source, which could be either human or non-human. The human instrument falls back on techniques such as interview (ranging from close-ended to open-ended to one-on-one, and including focus groups and web-based interactions), observation (from participant to non-participant), and non-verbal cues (Creswell 2007; Creswell and Poth 2017; Lincoln and Guba 1991). Non-human sources include unobtrusive measures, document and record analysis (from private to public), and audiovisual materials (from photographs to participant-created artifacts) (Creswell 2007; Creswell and Poth 2017; Lincoln and Guba 1991). New forms of data have emerged in recent years like texts from email messages, short and multimedia messages, living stories, metaphorical visual narratives, digital archives, autobiography, journals, field notes, letters, conversations, personal-family social artifacts (Creswell 2007), poems, music, sounds, ritual objects (Creswell and Poth 2017), and postings from social media (Patton 2015). A list of data types is presented in Table 3.1. A good qualitative researcher

Table 3.1 Types of data.

Human Sources	Non-Human Sources
Interviews	*Documents and Records*
One-on-one or focus groups	Field notes or journals
Structured (formal, focused, or standardized)	Personal: journals or diaries, letters, emails, private blogs
Unstructured (informal, in-depth, specialized, or exploratory)	Organizational: reports, strategic plans, charts, medical records
	Biographies, autobiographies
Storytelling	*Audiovisual*
Living stories	Video or film
Observation	Websites, tweets, Facebook messages, short and multimedia messages, digital archives
Complete participant	
Participant as observer	Sounds: music, car horns, childrens' laughter
Non-participant	Phone or computer-based messages
Complete observer	Metaphorical visual narratives
	Poems
	Ritual objects
	Personal-family social artifacts

employs rigorous data collection methods (Creswell and Poth 2017). Interviewing and observation are the two most commonly used methods in different qualitative research designs, including phenomenology, grounded theory, ethnography, narrative studies, and case study research.

3.3 Forms of Data

3.3.1 Interviewing

The interview is the favorite methodological tool of the qualitative researcher (Lincoln and Guba 1991). An interview is a conversation with a purpose. Denzin and Lincoln (1994) describe it as the art of asking and listening. Qualitative interviewing is motivated by the aim of eliciting information useful to a study. The interviewer in a qualitative research study enters the interviewee's world and perspectives, and wants them to talk about their internal states and tell their stories (Patton 2015), including obtaining here-and-now constructions of persons, events, organizations, feelings, motivations, claims, concerns, and other entities (Patton 2015). The research inquirer is a partner in information development, and the interviewing relationship is one of equals (Patton 2015).

Qualitative interviewing begins with the assumptions that the perspective of others is meaningful, knowable, and able to be made explicit (Lincoln and Guba 1991). A major advantage of interviews is that they permit the respondent to move back and forth in time – to reconstruct the past, interpret the present, and predict the future. Interviews are likely to provide a relatively complete and in-depth picture compared with other forms of inquiry (Guba and Lincoln 1981). They can be structured (formal, focused, or standardized) or unstructured (informal, in-depth, specialized, exploratory). The informal, in-depth, unstructured interview is the most open-ended approach (Patton 2015). In unstructured interviews, the phenomenon of interest is expected to emerge from the respondent's perception of the broad issues raised by the inquirer (Lincoln and Guba 1991). Questions emerge from the immediate context, and are asked in the natural course of things and the respondent's "natural language" (Guba and Lincoln 1981). There is no predetermination of questions or wordings (Patton 2015). This is the mode of choice in naturalistic inquiries when the interviewer does not know what the respondents know, and must therefore rely on their responses. Being unstructured does not mean that the interview is unfocused. Keeping in mind the phenomenon of interest, the research questions and the overall purpose of the inquiry inform the interview process, but the interviewer is free to go where the data and respondents lead (Patton 2015).

One-on-one interviews can be face-to-face (with or without the use of technology), by telephone, or in writing through text messaging or an online chat function. Focus group interviews can be done online, including via chat rooms and bulletin board groups (Creswell and Poth 2017). Creswell and Poth (2017) state: "Regardless of the interview mode, care must be taken to create an environment as comfortable as possible and, in group settings, to encourage all participants to talk and to monitor individuals who may

Table 3.2 Qualitative research design data collection techniques.

Phenomenology	Grounded Theory	Ethnography	Case Study	Narrative Research
Interviews with 5–30 people	Interviews with 20–30 people	Participant observations, interviews, artifacts and documents of a single culture-sharing group	Extensive forms, such as documents and records, interviews, observations, and physical artifacts for 1–4 cases	Notes, interview protocol

dominate the conversation" (p. 164). Weaknesses in unstructured interviewing include its inefficiency and cost, the inability to pre-test or standardize it, and the impossibility of replication, since the sole instrument of the study is the researcher. The interviewer can also influence the outcome of the interview through subtle cues they transmit, and possibly alienate the respondent by giving them the wrong kinds of cues (Guba and Lincoln 1981). Different qualitative inquiry traditions have varied interview methods and approaches, including the ethnographic, traditional social science, phenomenological, social constructionist, hermeneutic, narrative inquiry, and life-story interview. The data collection techniques from these different approaches are described in Table 3.2.

3.3.1.1 Phenomenological Interviews

Phenomenological interviewing involves an informal interactive process that aims to elicit a personal comprehensive description of a lived experience of a phenomenon (van Manen 1990, 2014; Patton 2015) for a small number of individuals who have experienced it. Phenomenologists gather other people's experiences because it allows them, in a vicarious sort of way, to become more experienced themselves (van Manen 2014). The focus of the interview is the direct description of a particular situation or event as it is lived through, without offering causal explanations or interpretive generalizations (Patton 2015). Phenomenological interviewing is less concerned with the factual accuracy than the plausibility of an account – whether it is true to our living sense of it. Qualitative inquiry – strategically, philosophically, and methodologically – aims to minimize the imposition of predetermined responses when gathering data (Lincoln and Guba 1991). Only broad-ranging questions are asked, so that the respondents can offer up testimony on their own terms (Guba and Lincoln 1989). Asking a truly open-ended question allows participants to respond in their own words, to determine what dimensions, themes, and images/words they will use to describe their thoughts, feelings, and experiences, and to select from a full repertoire of possible responses. Interview questions also center around meaning (What is the meaning of an experience?) and analogy (What is it like to experience?) (Morse 1994). The quality of the information obtained during an interview is largely dependent on the interviewer. There should be a genuine interest, an utmost respect for the perspectives of the interviewee, and appropriate interview skills and techniques (Lincoln and Guba 1991; Patton 2015).

Phenomenological interview and related methods are also used to gather pre-reflective experiential accounts (van Manen 2014). Van Manen (2014) emphasizes that it is extremely difficult to get interviewees to actually tell an experiential account in pre-reflective terms. It is much easier to get them to talk about an experience than to tell an experience as lived through. Experiential accounts or lived experience descriptions are never truly identical to the pre-reflective experiences themselves. All recollections, reflections, descriptions, and taped interviews about experiences or transcribed conversations are already transformations of those experiences. The procedures for preparing and conducting interviews are presented in Table 3.3.

Table 3.3 Procedures for preparing and conducting interviews.

1. Determine the open-ended questions to be answered.
2. Decide who to interview: identify interviewees using purposeful sampling; obtain an informed consent; determine where the interview will take place (a distraction-free place).
3. Prepare for the interview: distinguish and decide the type of interview based on mode and interactions; decide on an appropriate sequence of questions, even if the interview is unstructured; pilot test the interview, if it is the structured type; know your role, how to dress, and the level of formality; confirm the time and place of the interview ahead of time; ensure you have a working recording device and adequate recording procedures; plan for transcription procedures.
4. Begin the interview: reiterate the nature and purpose of the interview; ask "grand tour" questions; be clear; listen; provide a calm, relaxing atmosphere; allow the respondent time to organize their thoughts.
5. Pace the interview and keep it productive: maintain an easy rhythm and allow for "talk turn" pace; be flexible; use probes as appropriate; be both empathic and neutral; make transitions; watch for gestures and non-verbal cues; calls for examples and verifications; call for reactions and reformulations of what was said; call for more information; be prepared for the unexpected; be present throughout.
6. Terminate the interview and gain closure: summarize and play back; allow the respondent to add, subtract, or modify the data provided; thank the respondent for their participation and cooperation; remind the respondent about the details of any follow-up interviews, if planned.
7. After the interview: retire to a private room to write down notes and reflect on observations and non-verbal cues; get your notes in order for subsequent analysis; with a "fresh mind," listen to the audio-taped data a few times while checking the interview notes to reconstruct the interview process; prepare the audio-taped data for professional transcription; once the interview transcripts are obtained, listen again to the audio-taped data a few times while comparing against the transcripts; write notes in the margins of the transcripts to record any errors or corrections and any thoughts or recollection you may have; prepare the data for further triangulation (data and investigator) and member checking.

3.3.2 Storytelling

The life-story interview is another approach used to gather qualitative data within the phenomenological tradition through the storytelling process (Patton 2015). The participant can choose to tell the story of an event as it is lived. The resulting product is a first-person narrative – the essence of what has happened. It reveals how a specific human life is constructed and reconstructed in representing that life as a story (Patton 2015). Both interviewing and storytelling entail varied preparation and procedures, as described in Table 3.3.

Before a life-story interview, the qualitative researcher must ask the following questions: What are some of the things to keep in mind in conducting this interview? Where would be an appropriate place for the interview? What is the interactional sphere that contributes to the interview? What attitude is conducive for a successful interview? How should I conduct myself? (van Manen 2014). In interviewing and storytelling, the qualitative inquirer should observe instances in which non-verbal cues contrast with verbal reporting, which raise questions about truthfulness and completeness. Non-verbal cues can be used later as supplementary information on questionable items in the data that require more detailed attention. Thus, observation is vital in qualitative research data collection.

3.3.3 Observation

Observation is one of the most important methods for collecting data in qualitative research that provides in-depth, here-and-now experience. It is the act of noting a phenomenon through the five senses and recording it for scientific purposes (Creswell and Poth 2017). The researcher may watch physical settings, participants, activities, interactions, conversations, and their own behaviors during observation. A major purpose of observation is to see firsthand what is going on, rather than simply assuming that we know (Patton 2015). Naturalistic observations take place in the field, where the researcher observes and describes the meanings of what they perceive. Descriptions of observations should be factual, accurate, and thorough. For ethnographers, the field is the cultural setting. The value of a direct, personal contact with and observations of a setting through fieldwork is in allowing us to better understand and capture the context within which people interact.

Ethics demands that observations be overt and take place in a natural setting rather than a contrived one. A contrived context literally alters the phenomenon being studied in fundamental ways. Observing in a setting is a special skill, consisting of a series of procedural steps for preparing and conducting observations. These procedures are not the focus of this chapter. Observational data may be recorded in modes paralleling those available to the interviewer. Film or videotape recording is an example. There are four observation types: complete participant (researcher is fully engaged with the people being observed), participant as observer (researcher participates in activity at the site), non-participant or observer as participant (researcher is an outsider of the group under study), and complete observer (researcher is neither seen nor noticed by participants). An observational protocol can be used to record information (Creswell and Poth 2017).

3.4 Data Recording Procedures

Data recording modes are two dimensions namely fidelity, and structure. Fidelity is the ability of the investigators to reproduce exactly the data as they become evident to them in the field. According to Lincoln and Guba (1991), the greatest fidelity can be obtained using audio and video recording. In the different designs of qualitative research, the raw data are collected in an unstructured form such as tape or digital recordings or transcripts of conversations. One of the advantages of audio- or videotaping is the opportunity for subsequent analysis by independent observers (Mays and Pope 1995). Audio- and videotaping also provide an unimpeachable data source, assuring completeness and the opportunity to review as often as is necessary, including to note for non-verbal cues such as significant pauses, raised voices, and emotional outburst (Lincoln and Guba 1991). The disadvantages are the possibilities of mechanical failure and battery discharge. Right after the interview, the interviewer should listen to the recording a few times and review the field notes or journals so that items not noted are recalled. The audiotaped data must be transcribed by a professional transcriptionist, and the transcript must be checked by the interviewer to account for any errors. Finally, the information obtained from the interview should be subjected to triangulation and further member checking (Lincoln and Guba 1991). Interview transcripts, field notes, and observations provide a descriptive account of the study. It is the researcher who must make sense of the data collected, by exploring, describing, interpreting, and understanding them.

3.5 Data Analysis and Presentation

Analyzing text from multiple forms of data is challenging to qualitative researchers, especially novices and doctoral students. For new researchers, data analysis is probably the most mysterious aspect of the qualitative endeavor (Maxwell 2005). Data analysis in naturalistic inquiries consists of preparing and organizing the data, reducing the data into themes through a process of coding, condensing the codes, and representing the data in figures, tables, or discussion (Creswell and Poth 2017). The constructivist researcher's methods for data analysis are iterative, interactive hermeneutic, at times intuitive, and most certainly open. Guba and Lincoln (1989) state that these methods are "Far from being the 'easy way out' that undisciplined, lazy, ignorant or incompetent inquirers might choose, in contrast to the more rigorous, disciplined and demanding conventional approach" (p. 183). Creswell and Poth (2017) present general analysis procedures that are fundamental to all forms of qualitative research. These procedures are illustrated in Table 3.4.

In the early stages of the data analysis process, the researcher usually organizes the data into digital files and creates a file naming system so it can be easily located later. Securing the data for long-term storage is done in order to protect the confidentiality of information obtained from the participants. Following the organization of the data, the naturalistic inquirer continues the analysis by getting a sense of the whole database. The transcripts are read in their entirety several times in order to better understand them and make the interviews come alive, before breaking them into parts. Rapid reading

Table 3.4 Qualitative general data analysis procedures.

1. Taking notes while reading: writing notes in the margins of field notes; highlighting certain information.
2. Sketching reflective thinking: writing reflective messages.
3. Summarizing field notes: drafting a summary on field notes.
4. Working with words: making metaphors.
5. Identifying codes: abstract or concrete coding; writing codes and memos.
6. Reducing codes to themes: noting patterns and themes; identifying salient themes and patterned regularities.
7. Counting frequency of codes: noting relationships of concepts and variables.
8. Relating categories: contextualizing with the framework from literature.
9. Relating categories to analytic frameworks in the literature.
10. Creating a point of view: scenes, audience, readers.
11. Displaying and reporting data: creating a graph, figure, or picture of the framework; displaying findings in tables, graphs, diagrams, and figures; comparing and contrasting cases.

allows the researcher to approach the data in a new light. Notes and memos are written in the margins of the transcripts, and field notes are explored to identify and track major organizing ideas and to allow further synthesis that might lead to higher-level analytic meanings. Memos are short phrases, ideas, or key concepts that occur to the reader. Notes from observations are explored at this point, too. These processes afford credibility to the qualitative data analysis process and outcomes by uncovering information from the data sources. There is always a question over the use of computers in qualitative data analysis, because of their utility in facilitating tasks and increasing productivity for those savvy in their use. Patton (2015) asserts that computer programs can facilitate the work of analysis, but cannot provide the creativity and intelligence that make each qualitative analysis unique. Moreover, new software is constantly being developed. Analysis of qualitative data involves creativity, intellectual discipline, analytical rigor, and a great deal of hard work. The credibility of the researcher enhances the quality of the analysis. This pertains to the researcher's experience, competence, training and preparation, intellectual rigor, perceived trustworthiness, professional credibility, and philosophical beliefs or paradigm bases (Lincoln and Guba 1991).

3.5.1 Coding

After organizing, reading, and memoing, the next steps are to describe, classify, and interpret the data. Coding is the heart of qualitative data analysis (Creswell and Poth 2017). It involves making sense of the texts from interviews, observations, and documents. The process entails building detailed descriptions, applying codes, developing themes, and providing interpretations in the light of the researcher's own views and perspectives from the literature. Coding also involves aggregating the texts or visual data into small categories of information and assigning them a label. A list of tentative codes is made. Not all information from the transcripts is used in a qualitative study. Some data may be discarded (data reduction). Regardless of the size of the database,

Creswell and Poth (2017) recommend a final code list of no more than 25–30 categories of information, which can be reduced or combined into five of six themes or categories. Themes and categories in qualitative research are broad units of information that consist of several codes aggregated to form an idea. Some strategies for exploring and developing themes are: using memoing to capture emerging thematic ideas; highlighting noteworthy quotes as you code; creating diagrams representing relationships among codes or emerging concepts; drafting summary statements of recurring or striking aspects of the data; and focusing on the process of interpreting.

The researcher next tries to make sense of the data by making careful judgments about what is meaningful in the patterns, themes, and categories generated by the analysis and linking the interpretation to the larger research literature developed by others. Some questions that can be asked to guide the interpretation are: What surprising information did you not expect to find? What information is conceptually interesting or unusual to participants and the audience? What are the dominant interpretations, and what are the alternate notions? (p. 196) (Creswell and Poth 2017).

In the final phase, a diagram or figure is created to represent the relationships among concepts and themes, for use in the reporting of the study findings. There are specific coding procedures – developing and assessing interpretation techniques and representing and visualizing data methods – inherent to other naturalistic approaches, namely narrative research, phenomenology, grounded theory, ethnography, and case study. A summary of these procedures is presented in Tables 3.5–3.7.

3.5.2 Triangulation

Triangulation of data sources, theory, methodology, and the use of multiple analysts also contributes to quality data analysis (Denzin and Lincoln 1998). Triangulation as a technique for promoting the credibility of qualitative research was first advocated by Denzin in 1970. Denzin (1971) asserts that triangulation forces the observer to combine

Table 3.5 Classifying codes into themes in qualitative research designs.

Phenomenology	Grounded Theory	Ethnography	Case Study	Narrative Research
Describe personal experiences through epoche	Describe open coding categories	Describe the social setting, actors, and events	Describe the case and its content	Describe the patterns across the objective set of experiences
Describe the essence of the phenomenon	Select one open coding to build toward central phenomenon in process	Draw a picture of the event		Identify and describe the stories into a chronology

Source: Creswell, J. W. & Poth, C. N. (2017). *Qualitative Inquiry & Research Design: Choosing Among Five Approaches*, 4th ed., Sage Publications.

Table 3.6 Developing and assessing interpretations in qualitative research designs.

Phenomenology	Grounded Theory	Ethnography	Case Study	Narrative Research
Develop significant statements	Engage in axial coding – causal condition, context, intervening conditions, strategies, and consequences	Analyze data for themes and patterned regularities	Use categorical aggregation to establish themes or patterns	Locate epiphanies within stories
Group statements into meaning units	Develop the theory			Identify contextual materials

Source: Creswell, J. W. & Poth, C. N. (2017). *Qualitative Inquiry & Research Design: Choosing Among Five Approaches*, 4th ed., Sage Publications.

Table 3.7 Representing and visualizing the data in qualitative research designs.

Phenomenology	Grounded Theory	Ethnography	Case Study	Narrative Research
Develop a textural description "what happened"	Engage in selective coding and interrelate categories to develop a "story" or propositions or matrix	Interpret and make sense of the findings – "how the culture works"		Use direct interpretation
Develop a structural description – "how the phenomenon was experienced"				Develop naturalistic generalizations of what was "learned"
Develop the "essence" using a composite description				

Source: Creswell, J. W. & Poth, C. N. (2017). *Qualitative Inquiry & Research Design: Choosing Among Five Approaches*, 4th ed., Sage Publications.

multiple data sources, research methods, and theoretical schemes. It is done to reduce the likelihood of misinterpretation; thus, various procedures are employed, like redundancy of data gathering and procedural challenges to explanations, using multiple perceptions to clarify meaning, and verifying the repeatability of an observation or interpretation (Denzin and Lincoln 1998). Triangulation strategies reduce the risk that the researcher's conclusion will reflect only the systematic biases or limitations of a specific source or method, and allow one to gain a broader understanding and more secure understanding of the issues under investigation (Maxwell 2005). Webb et al. (1966) state that triangulation, although difficult, is very much worth doing, because it makes data and findings credible.

Triangulation of data is crucially important in naturalistic studies. The process involves corroborating evidence from different sources to shed light on a theme or perspective. It is also about comparing and cross-checking the consistency of information derived at different times and by different means from interviews, observations, and documents (Patton 2015). Denzin (1978) identifies four types of triangulation: data, investigator, theory, and methodological triangulation. This section focuses on data and investigator triangulation. As a study unfolds, and significant information emerge, steps should be taken to validate each against at least one other source (e.g., a second interview) and/or a second method (e.g., an observation in addition to an interview) (Lincoln and Guba 1991). This is called data triangulation. If the data gathered from different sources are found to be consistent, the credibility of the study is promoted (Schmidt and Brown 2015). Richer descriptions of phenomena thus result (Seale 1999), and the validity and accuracy of the findings are improved (Creswell and Poth 2017). Investigator triangulation is the use of several researchers or evaluators to independently analyze the same qualitative data and compare their findings (Denzin 1978; Patton 2015).

3.6 Data Collection, Analysis, and Presentation, Challenges, Tips, and the Importance of a Mentor

Conducting qualitative research is a complex, tedious, and difficult endeavor, especially for novices and doctoral students. The guidance of an expert and patient mentor is needed to help the mentee pivot on the long and challenging journey of completing the study. The experiences of doctoral students also vary. While some gain a quality doctoral experience with exemplary mentoring and socialization, others do not receive the coaching and preparation they need to succeed in their research projects. Students must carefully and wisely choose a dissertation chair who will willingly and thoughtfully guide them throughout the process of intellectual inquiry. The role of the mentor or chair includes offering constructive and critical advising and honest support, acting as a role model, giving timely feedback, maintaining an effective dialogue, having regular contact (face-to-face or via email, telephone, or technology like Skype or Zoom), allowing open negotiations of responsibilities, maximizing the professional and personal potential of the mentee, and being a source of emotional support, encouragement, and affirmation.

Although doctoral students learn about the data collection process in their research methodology coursework and are supervised by their dissertation committee chair, they still experience challenges and unanticipated occurrences during data collection and analysis as they embark on the intense and demanding work of a qualitative study. First is the question of what mode of data collection to use, and what to do in terms of timing, duration, and location/setting (environment). Issues can arise related to human subject participation in interviews, observation, or focus groups, such as choosing and locating participants, lack of willingness, rapport, and concerns about the confidentiality of information and privacy. Researcher challenges include how to dress for the interview, lack of confidence, lack of experience in starting, conducting, and maintaining a comfortable and fruitful interaction (including dealing with "sensitive topics") and the complex tasks of analyzing and interpreting data.

Early-career researchers and doctoral students should be mentored on how to address the challenges encountered during data collection. The location chosen for an interview should be neutral, and convenient and safe for both participant and researcher. Qualitative data collection should be conducted in a naturalistic environment that allows participants to freely express themselves while preserving their privacy and confidentiality of information. Participants should also have the free choice to participate or not in the data collection process, and should be allowed to withdraw at any point if they so wish.

Before each interview, "icebreakers" should be incorporated to make the interviewee feel at ease. It can become difficult to delve deeper into a respondent's thoughts when a specific area of the phenomenon becomes "sensitive." It is important to re-engage and re-focus by taking time and allowing the interviewee to gain a grasp of the last thought they expressed. Researcher fatigue should be avoided. Conducting back-to-back interviews is overwhelming. Early-career researchers should limit the number of interviews they conduct in a single day. One or two a day, lasting 45–60 minutes, should be enough. They should also allow themselves 30–60 minutes between interviews to reflect, write notes, decompress, and have a debriefing with a colleague or advisor.

3.7 Conclusion

This chapter presented several components of data collection, analysis, and representation. It began by attending to ethical considerations, including around gaining access to and building rapport at the research site, protecting the rights of the participants by gaining institutional review board approval, and purposeful sampling. It described the data collection procedures of interviewing, storytelling, and observation, including approaches to recording information and proper storage of databases. Further, it presented data management and organization approaches including reading, memoing, identifying, and classifying codes into themes, developing interpretations, and representing data visually. Finally, it examined the challenges that early-career researchers and novices encounter and made recommendations for addressing them.

References

Creswell, J.W. (2007). *Qualitative Inquiry and Research Design: Choosing among Five Approaches*, 2e. Sage Publications.

Creswell, J.W. and Poth, C.N. (2017). *Qualitative Inquiry & Research Design: Choosing Among Five Approaches*, 4e. Sage Publications.

Denzin, N.K. (1970). *The Research Act in Sociology*, 1e. Butterworth.

Denzin, N.K. (1971). The logic of naturalistic inquiry. *Social Forces* 50 (2): 166–182.

Denzin, N.K. (1978). *The Research Act: A Theoretical Introduction to Sociological Methods*, 2e. McGraw-Hill.

Denzin, N.K. and Lincoln, Y.S. (1994). *Handbook of Qualitative Research*. Sage Publications.

Denzin, N.K. and Lincoln, Y.S. (1998). *Strategies of Qualitative Inquiry*. Sage Publications.

Devers, K.J. and Frankel, R.M. (2014). Study design in qualitative research – 2: sampling and data collection strategies. *Education for Health* 13 (2): 263–271.

Guba, E.G. and Lincoln, Y.S. (1981). *Effective Evaluation*. Jossey-Bass.

Guba, E.G. and Lincoln, Y.S. (1989). *Fourth Generation Evaluation*. Sage Publications.

Lincoln, Y.S. and Guba, E.G. (1991). *Naturalistas Inquiry*. Sage Publications.

Maxwell, J.A. (2005). *Qualitative Research Design: An Interactive Approach*, 2e. Sage Publications.

Mays, N. and Pope, C. (1995). Rigour and qualitative research. *BMJ* 311: 109–112.

Morse, J.M. (1994). *Critical Issues in Qualitative Research Methods*. Sage Publications.

Patton, M.Q. (2015). *Qualitative Evaluation and Research Methods*, 4e. Sage Publications.

Schmidt, N.A. and Brown, J. (2015). *Evidence-Based Practice for Nurses: Appraisal and Application of Research*, 3e. Jones and Bartlett.

Seale, C. (1999). *The Quality of Qualitative Research*. Sage Publications.

van Manen, M. (1990). *Researching Lived Experience: Human Science for an Action Sensitive Pedagogy*. State University of New York Press.

van Manen, M. (2014). *Phenomenology of Practice: Meaning-Giving Methods in Phenomenological Research and Writing*. Left Coast Press.

Webb, E.J., Campbell, D.T., Schwartz, R.D., and Seches, L. (1966). *Unobtrusive Measures: Non-reactive Research in the Social Sciences*. Rand McNally.

4

Data Analysis Software in Qualitative Research

Qualitative researchers are increasingly using software for qualitative data analysis. Initially, naturalistic inquirers as a social movement had a radical response to the use of computers for statistical work. There was a heartfelt rejection of this technological advancement as it conveyed dehumanization, over-control, and obsession with technology.

4.1 Brief Historical Overview of the Use of Software in Qualitative Research

The use of computers for basic content analysis of text became popular in the humanities from the 1960s onwards. Social researchers explained the advantages of computers for data analysis, but they were largely confined to statistical undertakings until the 1980s, when qualitative researchers began to catch up (Silverman 2005). A plethora of software was produced in this decade, but mainly designed for librarians, executives, and banks (Richards and Richards 1994). The 1990s ushered in a small group of programs designed for specific approaches to qualitative inquiries, but they were difficult to access and not professionally "user-friendly" (Richards and Richards 1994). Many qualitative researchers remained distanced from this innovation because of feelings that it might impose an alien logic on their analytic procedures (Silverman 2005). Discussions and debates continued about the assumption that qualitative data analysis software (**QDAS**) would improve research. Indeed, unsubstantiated and outdated criticisms of QDAS persist to this day. Consequently, there are practical concerns over how various software programs and computer-based analytical and data management applications should be used, as well as issues over the fact that some inquirers treat the software as the method of analysis (Jackson et al. 2018).

Reviewing all of the programs that are currently available or seeking to describe the finer details of how particular packages work is not the aim of this chapter. Information about this technology becomes out of date quickly, since software developers continue to release new product versions and features. Qualitative studies have flourished, and a number of them are conducted by novices, early-career researchers, and experienced investigators. Conducting a qualitative inquiry is a difficult and time-consuming endeavor in itself. Additionally, the use of computer-assisted qualitative data analysis software (**CAQDAS**) in these investigations presents some challenges to both the beginner and the expert alike.

4.2 To Use or Not to Use Qualitative Data Analysis Software?

Computer programs developed to organize data for qualitative analysis have been available since 1984. Woods et al. (2016) found that the number of researchers reporting use of QDAS was increasing. The majority of studies using ATLAS.ti and NVivo are published in health sciences journals by authors from the United Kingdom, United States, Netherlands, Canada, and Australia. They also articulated that the vast majority of naturalistic inquirers use QDAS for data management and analysis, with fewer using it for data collection/creation or to visually display their methods and findings. Software is one means of rigorously combing data for the analyst/researcher in search of insight within an environment where the data are complex and typically based on large, potentially subjunctivized data sets (Atherton and Elsmore 2007). Although QDAS is seen increasingly as an "enabling technology," acceptance of software-based data analysis protocols for qualitative research has not been universal (Atherton and Elsmore 2007). Debates still continue over the use of QDAS (Hinchliffe and Crang 1997; Kelle 1996; Mangabeira 1996; Miles and Weitzman 1996; Morison and Moir 1998; Webb 1999). In an appraisal of the Sociological Abstracts database, MacMillan and Koenig (2004) found 31 references to Nud*ist, Atlas.ti, NVivo, winMAX, Kwalitan, MAXqda, Qualrus, or Hyperresearch since 1990, compared to 220 references to SPSS, SAS, and Stata (all quantitative software). Why is this so?

QDAS enables efficient handling and management of large data sets, thus taking away this hard work from the researcher. Other advantages include being freed from manual and clerical tasks, saving time, increasing flexibility, and improving validity and auditability (St. John and Johnson 2000). In spite of these positive effects, QDAS approaches have been found to be more time-costly than other methods of data coding and analysis, and yet have not generated superior results. The application of simple quantification techniques such as key word counts and hierarchical coding does not adequately address the ambiguities of social interaction or context-dependent meaning sets (Atherton and Elsmore 2007). There are also concerns that QDAS use is an increasingly deterministic and rigid process, that it requires increasing amounts of time and energy to be spent on learning new packages and programs, and that it leads to increased commercialism, distraction from the real work of analysis, and increased emphasis on the volume and breadth of data rather than on depth and meaning (St. John and Johnson 2000).

4.3 What Is Qualitative Data Analysis Software?

QDAS provides tools that help with qualitative research such as transcription analysis, coding, text interpretation, recursive abstraction, content and discourse analysis, and grounded theory methodology. It is used in healthcare, legal, sociology, anthropology, music, geography, geology, forensics, tourism, criminology, marketing, education, theology, philosophy, history, market research, focus group analysis, and most other fields using qualitative approaches. A number of top QDAS applications are summarized in Table 4.1.

CAQDAS Networking Project at the University of Surrey was established as a focal point for discussions about QDAS programs in 1994. This chapter will specifically focus on CAQDAS, citing studies using ATLAS.ti or NVivo because they are two of the longest used QDAS tools (Muhr 1991; Woods et al. 2016).

4.4 Computer-Assisted Qualitative Data Analysis Software

CAQDAS can be helpful in doing qualitative data analysis, but it also has its limitations (Silverman 2005). The main advantages are speed of handling large volumes of data; improvement of rigor, including the production of counts of phenomena and searching for deviant cases; facilitation of team research, including the development of coding schemes; and help with sampling decisions, be they in the service of representativeness or to allow theory development (Silverman 2005).

4.4.1 Advantages

4.4.1.1 Speed

Qualitative research is a lengthy process that an effective data management software package can significantly help to expedite (St. John and Johnson 2000). This saves time and effort, which might be otherwise spent on boring clerical work involving mounds of photocopied paper, color-coded, sorted into piles, cut up, pasted, and so on. This in turn give analysts more time to think about the meaning of data, enabling rapid feedback on the results of a particular analytic idea so that new ones can be formulated (Silverman 2005). Silverman (2005) states: "Qualitative analysis then becomes more devoted to creative and intellectual tasks, less immersed in routine" (p. 190).

4.4.1.2 Rigor

CAQDAS can help researchers demonstrate that their conclusions are based on rigorous analysis (Silverman 2005). One important feature is the way it enables all data related to

Table 4.1 Types of qualitative data analysis software.

Qualitative Data Analysis Software	Research Use
Nvivo	Qualitative and mixed methods
ATLAS.ti	Qualitative (leading software; most powerful and intuitive)
MAXQDA	Qualitative, quantitative, and mixed Methods for Windows and Mac OS
Quirkos	Qualitative
WebQDA	Qualitative (collaborative and distributed environment)
Dedoose	Qualitative (has the best encryption)
HyperRESEARCH	Qualitative (has cross-platform capabilities)
Raven's Eye	Natural language analysis tool based on quantitative phenomenology
Qiqqa	Research and reference manager to read and annotate pdfs
Focuss On	Allows users to conduct online interviews and text analysis without the involvement of an external agency (chat)
F4analyze	Interpretation of qualitative data on Windows, Mac OS, and Linux in the context of grounded theory, qualitative text analysis, and documentary and other interpretive methods; allows the recording of memos in text passages and the writing of comments on texts and codes
Annotations	New solution for Mac OS; makes adding and managing notes to text simpler; allows the ability to highlight texts with colors, assign custom keywords, or quickly add notes of any size.
Datagrav	Presents server and cloud platforms and integration modules for interacting with IT infrastructure.
QDA Miner	Leader in text analysis, with qualitative, quantitative, and mixed methods programs.
Saturate App	Qualitative: analyzes text and audio files, in which a user's own codes can be created; useful for team projects, allowing multiple team members to contribute to coding interview transcripts; allows coding to be exported as CSV files, which can be imported into a spreadsheet.

a topic to be examined, as opposed to the human tendency of privileging parts that fit with one's own assumptions and worldviews (St. John and Johnson 2000). All materials are coded, can be retrieved, and are unlikely to be lost. Software enables the management of data collection and analysis, and so is an enabler of qualitative research that is rigorous in the sense that it increases the ability to extract insights from data by ordering it in more searchable and manipulable forms and formats (Atherton and Elsmore 2007).

Some qualitative researchers do not make their analytical strategies explicit. CAQDAS will help make strategies visible, thereby providing a basis for credibility and validity by making available an audit trail that can be scrutinized (St. John and Johnson 2000).

4.4.1.3 Team Research

CAQDAS can support collaborative team-based analyses in which several researchers analyze a data set involving multiple analysts coding the same data and then integrating their coding. For some research teams, one researcher is primarily responsible for coding while others code a sample to check for accuracy and validity. Some teams also report using collaborative analysis to inductively develop codes and coding rules that they then use to analyze the remainder of the data. The current versions of ATLAS.ti (v. 7) and NVivo (v. 10) support collaborative analyses by recording and tracking which researchers have added codes to the data, thus making it possible to identify coders later when files are merged (Woods et al. 2016).

4.4.1.4 Sampling

CAQDAS allows for encouragement of consistent coding and avoidance of anecdotalism (Silverman 2005). The rapid retrieval that CAQDAS makes possible can help in dealing with larger samples, thus enhancing the confidence with which empirical generalizations are made. However, in qualitative research, developing a theory is the aim, rather than generality (e.g., comparing cases where a phenomenon exists with those where it does not, seeing which other conditions appear to be associated with a phenomenon). This strategy is called constant comparison, as described in grounded theory. CAQDAS can help with this by ensuring that comparison of cases is systematic rather than impressionistic. It can rapidly indicate which cases show a phenomenon, as well as what other conditions are present in each case (Silverman 2005).

4.4.2 Disadvantages

4.4.2.1 Word Processing

Most CAQDAS programs require data to be entered in a word-processing package, which the analyst must read and code. This remains one of the most time-consuming elements of qualitative data analysis, which computers do not remove. The time-saving elements of CAQDAS occur at the later stage of data search and retrieval. The cost of moving from a word processor is not a strong argument, since CAQDAS programs are less expensive than the most statistical software, like SPSS (Silverman 2005).

4.4.2.2 Narrow Approach to Analysis

CAQDAS software generally provides value for organization, and allows retrieval of content rather than discovery of form or structure. For discourse analysts and semioticians, CAQDAS would be pointless in the detailed analysis of short data extracts, and would not substitute for in-depth consideration of the meaning of particular, telling instances. It also does not support analysis of the formal structure of narratives, except in the case of ETHNO software (Silverman 2005).

Atherton and Elsmore (2007) – both QDAS users and experts – used a structured debate in the form a narrative dialogue in discussing the pros and cons, benefits and pitfalls of the use of CAQDAS. They assert that qualitative research requires the extraction of extensive amounts of data from personal interactions between researcher and subject, and so is a complex, socialized dynamic set, occurring within a social context. The risk with using standardized software packages is that they do not stimulate, or drive, consideration of where the researcher is "coming from," and so do not provide a means of dealing with the subjectivity and agenda of the researcher in a reflexive way. There is a concern that standardized formats for data analysis and presentation are based on generic rather than tailored approaches to data organization and presentation. The issue is the genericization of data analysis. Atherton and Elsmore (2007) state: "Using generic software protocols, particularly when repeated regularly, creates an epistemological 'comfort blanket' for researchers, in that they produce an expected and defined approach to dealing with data (again regardless of context)" (p. 67).

Qualitative research seeks to address the context within which a subject operates. It attempts to deal with the ways in which data are de-contextualized, and to preserve as much as possible of the context, its significance for insight, and its meaning. Research, in other words, de-contextualizes, and so distorts and changes the original. Software-based qualitative data analysis places extracted data in a new context, and hence removes much of their meaning. How we deal with meaning in and out of context lies at the heart of the research process, and provides an underpinning rationale for undertaking qualitative research. All research methods remove data from their situ and embedded meaning (Atherton and Elsmore 2007; St. John and Johnson 2000). The basis for undertaking qualitative research is to explore "thick" rich data for meanings, conceptual understanding, and discourses (St. John and Johnson 2000).

There is also an issue around homogenizing qualitative data analysis approaches. The use of software makes the researcher structure the data before they are entered in the computer, thus making the analysis rigid and inflexible, or like a "straight-jacket." This assumes that the data are textual, but there are other forms of data too, like photographs, maps, brochures, films, audiotapes, videotapes, diagrams, organizational charts, music, paintings, drawings, objects, and artifacts (St. John and Johnson 2000).

4.4.2.3 Small Data Extracts

For researchers and conversation analysts interested in reading and re-reading a short extract from a talk, or a single paragraph of text, there is no point in using CAQDAS. Such analysis can easily be done manually. After all, one of the biggest advantages of CAQDAS is its speed of handling large volumes of data. CAQDAS programs are also advanced and have theory-driven modes of qualitative analysis that can be extended by the comparative analysis of different data extracts (Silverman 2005).

4.5 Two of the Current Top Mainstream Software Packages

There are many sources that discuss the current top mainstream software packages. It is best in this regard to explore relevant internet sites rather than books, because new program versions are continually emerging. There are also online discussions about such packages, as well as blogs from developers who want consumers around the world to engage in a conversation related to the use, issues, usability, and other related matters concerning their software packages. Two very common and widely-used packages – ATLAS.ti and NVivo – will be presented here in order to illustrate what these innovations can offer to researchers in terms of qualitative data analysis, allowing them to choose the package that best suits their needs.

Woods et al. (2016) conducted a content analysis of 763 empirical articles published in the Scopus database between 1994 and 2013, exploring how researchers use the ATLAS.ti and NVivo QDAS programs. They found that the top four countries for ATLAS.ti use were the United States, United Kingdom, Netherlands, and Canada, while the top four countries for NVivo were the United States, United Kingdom, Australia, and Canada. NVivo originated from Australia, which may explain the relatively high number of articles from Australian authors. ATLAS.ti originated from Germany, but there are nonetheless very few studies published by Germans. The authors attribute this to their focus on English-language publications. For ATLAS.ti, the most frequently cited types of studies were interviews (32.1%), followed by focus groups (21.2%), grounded theory (12.9%), generic qualitative (8.3%), and ethnographic or observational studies (8%). For NVivo, it was generic "qualitative studies" (36.2%), thematic analysis/qualitative content analysis (15.2%), grounded theory (13.3%), focus group (9.7%), and interviews (8.5%). Researchers also reported using ATLAS.ti and NVivo to support three phases of the research process: data collection/creation, data analysis/management, and data display/representation of findings. Data analysis and management was the most frequently mentioned use, with 99.6% of studies using the software for this purpose (Woods et al. 2016).

Questions to ask and consider when choosing a QDAS package are presented in Table 4.2.

4.5.1 ATLAS.ti

ATLAS.ti is a software workbench that helps researchers perform qualitative analysis on large amounts of text, graphics, audio, or video. The program supports a wide range of data formats, including most common text formats (.txt, .do, .docx, and .pdf), "dozens" of graphic and audio formats (including .wav and .mp3), and many common video formats. One can also import data from Twitter or Evernote, surveys, or a reference manager. ATLAS.ti allows users to code, link, and visualize the data. Some of its unique features include an interactive margin area and a quotation-level tool that offers an analytic level below coding and better supports inductive, interpretive research approaches like grounded theory, hermeneutics, discourse analysis, sociology

Table 4.2 Considerations when choosing a qualitative data analysis software package.

- ▣ Do I know the capabilities of the packages that are available? (If not, where do I get advice?)
- ▣ Do I have the resources to purchase appropriate software and hardware and to prepare data for analysis?
- ▣ Do I know how to use the selected package? (If not, do I have access to education and help or customer support?)
- ▣ What are the advantages and disadvantages of this package to my research?
- ▣ What time and effort will be required if I use this package?
- ▣ What purpose will this package serve for this research project?
- ▣ Will this package handle the type of data I intend to collect?
- ▣ How do I intend to use this package?
- ▣ Will this package enable flexible handling of data for this research?
- ▣ Will this package enable me to interact with and reduce the data in a way that is consistent with my methods?
- ▣ Will this package maintain my data in context?
- ▣ What processes will I use to ensure that I maintain methodological integrity while using this package?
- ▣ Have I reviewed, corrected, and interacted with my data before entering it into the computer for analysis?

Source: St. John, W. & Johnson, P. (2000). The pros and cons of data analysis software for qualitative research. *Journal of Nursing Scholarship*, 32(4): 393–394.

of knowledge, and phenomenology (ATLAS.ti 2018). It also offers more extended features for theory development, including the capacity to create conceptual diagrams showing links between emerging ideas. These diagrams are themselves linked to instances of data, meaning that quotations illustrating theoretical statements can be gathered quickly (Silverman 2005).

4.5.2 NVivo

NVivo is the most used qualitative and mixed-methods data analysis software tool among academics and professional researchers globally. The program allows users to organize, store, and retrieve data, making work more efficient, saving time, and enabling one to rigorously back up findings with evidence. It also allows users to import data from virtually any source, including text, audio, video, emails, images, spreadsheets, online surveys, social media, and web content. More specifically, it stores and sorts data on one platform, from quantifiable demographic information to qualitative open-ended questions and interviews. It automatically sorts sentiment, themes, and attributes in seconds. It quickly exchanges data with SPSS for further statistical analysis. It easily cross-tabulates mixed-methods data and visualizes the results in order to allow brainstorming and mapping ideas, exploration of connections between project items, and discovery of new paths of investigation (NVivo 2018).

4.6 Challenges in the Use of CAQDAS, and the Importance of Training and a Mentor

There are continuous concerns, problems, and misunderstandings among both developers and researchers (novice and experts alike) about the use of software programs in qualitative analysis. Underuse is evident even today because users with little background in qualitative methods are likely to be unaware of the criteria for analytic adequacy (Mangabeira et al. 2004). There is a basic uncertainty over what software can and cannot do, the intricacies of the software program, the time and labor involved in learning how to operate it, and the perplexing jargon of the program-specific technical language describing its various functions (Macmillan and Koenig 2004). Another danger is the assumption that the software is the methodology, and that by simply learning how to operate the program, the researcher is doing analysis (Macmillan and Koenig 2004). Thus, appreciation of the qualitative method becomes effectively defined by the nature of the software used. Such descriptions create the impression that analysis is actually done by the software. This view also implies that the better the researcher is at working the program, the better the analysis (Macmillan and Koenig 2004). Researchers should be aware that QDAS is a tool for organizing data, not a method of analysis. It provides an alternative, complementary way of looking at data (Atherton and Elsmore 2007). CAQDAS packages vary in their approach to analysis and analytic procedures. Inquirers who have little background in qualitative analysis may think that the uncertainty must be an intrinsic characteristics of qualitative research (Mangabeira et al. 2004). It is therefore important that novices grasp the basic premises of qualitative analysis before they experiment with software. Some developers encourage caution in promoting software use, whereas others see education and better training as the main solutions.

Counter to the underuse of software in qualitative analysis is the belief that software packages are the only way to go in conducting qualitative research (Macmillan and Koenig 2004). CAQDAS is not a "universal" solution that is suitable for all qualitative research designs. Every naturalistic inquirer needs a clear and explicit rationale and reason for its use. The use of programs should be considered within the epistemological framework of the qualitative research design chosen to fit the study (Macmillan and Koenig 2004). Phenomena and research questions are defined not by the software tool but by the problems to be examined. The use of QDAS is "contingent" and "conditional" on the research question and its approach. All research methods are flawed and incomplete in one way or another (Atherton and Elsmore 2007). The question then is not what are the weaknesses of software packages, but what are their limitations in comparison with other approaches? Software users argue that the use of software protocols should be a complementary, and so valid, approach to organizing, examining, and understanding data. There should not be a sole reliance on programs as the only means of data analysis (Atherton and Elsmore 2007).

There are other controversies around the use of CAQDAS, like separation/distancing criticism (barriers between the researcher and the data may limit the researcher's ability to become close to and familiar with the data), homogenization/standardizing criticism (the theoretical preferences of the software developers and the way they display sample projects may facilitate a trend toward homogenization of method), mechanization/dehumanizing criticism (an overreliance on mechanization and systematization may lead to their being mistaken as markers of rigor), and quantification/decontextualizing criticism (computers may encourage postures of data extraction via coding, counting, and hypothesis testing at the expense of building qualitative interpretations and constructing theory) (Jackson et al. 2018). There is a risk that context and situated meaning are not communicated or transferred through the research process, and that this loss of contextualization of insight removes significance from findings (Atherton and Elsmore 2007).

In spite of all the criticisms presented in the literature, Jackson et al. (2018) state: "there are interesting, new experiences, made available to [us] by QDAS that contradict the short-sighted and perhaps technophobic criticisms about separation/distancing" (p. 85). The benefits of the use of software packages are: speed of handling of large volumes of data; improvement of rigor, including the production of counts of phenomena and searching for deviant cases; facilitation of team research, including the development of coding schemes; and help with sampling decisions as previously discussed (Silverman 2005). There is, however, clearly a need for more than practical training. Many researchers using CAQDAS have little training in social science methods (Macmillan and Koenig 2004). For users with less experience of the diversity of qualitative methods, texts describing CAQDAS as a method can perpetuate misunderstandings about the extent to which software functions produce analysis (Macmillan and Koenig 2004). Researchers should not be so infatuated with technology that it drives the research; instead, it should serve the research (St. John and Johnson 2000). Often, inquirers invest much money and time in learning to use a software package, and just when they believed they have mastered that particular program, developers produce new and improved versions (St. John and Johnson 2000). Diversity, creativity, new ideas, and innovation are encouraged in qualitative research and methodology; thus, investigators should conduct studies on the basis of the phenomenon or research question, purpose, and methods. The use of CAQDAS should not be an automatic assumption for every qualitative research endeavor. Qualitative data analysis can still be, and is, done manually.

Manual coding in data analysis is still often used by qualitative researchers. Good qualitative analysis is well-founded on traditional methods, and relies on good analytic work by a careful human researcher, in the same way that good writing is not guaranteed by the use of a word processor. When using manual coding, one can utilize folders and filing cabinets instead of computer-based directories and files to gather together materials that are examples of similar themes or analytic ideas. Manual methods of coding in qualitative data analysis, such as marking up selected text with codes, generating reports, and searching for key terms and usages, are labor-intensive, time-consuming, error-prone, and outdated, and yet are still preferred by some who are less familiar with computer-based software. It is these tasks that the computer can usefully assist with. However, the conceptual aspects of analysis, including reading the text, interpreting it, creating coding schemes, identifying fruitful searches, and making reports, require a human, and cannot be done by machines. Additionally, two factors to consider when choosing computer-assisted qualitative data analysis are the training and time required to master the software program and cost considerations. Moreover, it is important to have approval from a dissertation supervisor before applying any specific QDAS. In any case, both manual coding and the use of computerized software require a supervisor and a mentor who can assist the novice investigator undertake the complex, laborious process of data management and analysis.

4.7 Conclusion

It is clear that the introduction of computer-assisted data analysis software has expanded the ways in which qualitative researchers can collect, manage, and analyze data. This chapter looked at the role of software in qualitative inquiries, with some focus on the methodological issues surrounding program use, and identified the factors leading to the unrealistic expectation that the program is the methodology. It discussed the advantages and disadvantages of the use of CAQDAS in qualitative research, and provided a brief review of two very common and widely-used QDAS packages, ATLAS.ti and Nvivo. Software cannot always accomplish every research goal, and the researcher must remain in charge of the data analysis – not the other way around. The expertise, experience, and integrity of the inquirer must be considered in choosing the tools to use, giving respect to the research question, purpose, design, and methods. Those who have avoided the use of QDAS may need to start to confront the pleasures and pains of this technology. A healthy critique and debate about the impact of CAQDAS should continue, and developers' and users' ideas should be discussed and shared. Such openness and communication might help address the disagreements and criticisms related to CAQDAS use. Finally, having and making good use of a qualitative inquiry supervisor or mentor is beneficial for students, novices, and early career researchers in guiding them toward the completion of their endeavor.

References

Atherton, A. and Elsmore, P. (2007). Structuring qualitative enquiry in management and organization research: a dialogue on the merits of using software for qualitative data analysis qualitative research in organizations and management. Qualitative Research in Organization and Management International Journal 2 (1): 62–77.

ATLAS.ti Qualitative Data Analysis. (2018). What is ATLAS.ti? Available from https://atlasti.com/product/what-is-atlas-ti (accessed May 10, 2021).

Hinchliffe, S. and Crang, M. (1997). Software for qualitative research: 2. Some thoughts on "aiding" analysis. Environment and Planning: A: Economy and Space 29 (6): 109–125.

Jackson, K., Paulus, T., and Woolf, N.H. (2018). The walking dead genealogy: unsubstantiated criticisms of qualitative data analysis software (QDAS) and the failure to put them to rest. The Qualitative Report 23: 74–91.

Kelle, U. (1996). Computer-assisted qualitative data analysis in Germany. Current Sociology 44: 2225–2241.

Macmillan, K. and Koenig, T. (2004). The wow factor: preconceptions and expectations for data analysis software in qualitative research. Social Science Computer Review 22 (2): 179–186.

Mangabeira, W. (1996). CAQDAS and its diffusion across four countries: national specificities and common themes. Current Sociology 44: 191–205.

Mangabeira, W.C., Lee, R.M., and Feilding, N.G. (2004). Computers and qualitative research: adoption, use and representation. Social Science Computer Review 22 (2): 167–178.

Miles, M.B. and Weitzman, E. (1996). The state of qualitative data analysis software: what do we need? Current Sociology 44: 206–224.

Morison, M. and Moir, J. (1998). The role of computer software in the analysis of qualitative data: efficient clerk, research assistants or Trojan horse? Journal of Advanced Nursing 28 (1): 106–116.

Muhr, T. (1991). ATLAS/ti – a prototype for the support of text interpretation. Qualitative Sociology 14: 349–371.

NVivo. (2018). What is NVivo? Available from http://www.qsrinternational.com/nvivo/what-is-nvivo (accessed May 10, 2021).

Richards, T.J. and Richards, L. (1994). Using computers in qualitative research. In: Handbook of Qualitative Research (eds. N.K. Denzin and Y.S. Lincoln), 273–285. Sage Publications.

Silverman, D. (2005). Doing Qualitative Research, 2e. Sage Publications.

St. John, W. and Johnson, P. (2000). The pros and cons of data analysis software for qualitative research. Journal of Nursing Scholarship 32 (4): 393–394.

Webb, C. (1999). Analysing qualitative data: computerized and other approaches. Journal of Advance Nursing 29 (2): 323–330.

Woods, M., Paulus, T., Atkins, D.P., and Macklin, R. (2016). Advancing qualitative research using qualitative data analysis software (QDAS)? Reviewing potential versus practice in published studies using ATLAS.ti and NVivo, 1994–2013. Social Science Computer Review 34 (5): 597–617.

Enhancing the Rigor and Validity of Phenomenological Research

5

Rigor or Reliability and Validity in Qualitative Research
A Reconceptualization

onducting a naturalistic inquiry is in general not an easy task. Qualitative studies are more complex in many ways than traditional investigations. Quantitative research follows a structured, rigid, pre-set design, with the methods all prescribed. In naturalistic inquiries, planning and implementation are simultaneous, and the research design is emergent or may change. Preliminary steps must be accomplished before the design is fully implemented – from making initial contact and gaining entry to site to negotiating consent, building and maintaining trust, and identifying participants. The steps of a qualitative inquiry are repeated multiple times during the process. As the design unfolds, its elements are put into place; the inquirer has minimal control over the process and must be flexible. There is continuous reassessment and reiteration. Data collection is carried out using multiple techniques, and whatever the source may be, it is the researcher who is the sole instrument of the study and the primary mode of collecting the information. All the while during these processes, the qualitative inquirer must be concerned with rigor (Lincoln and Guba 1985). Appropriate activities must be carried out to ensure that rigor had been attended to in the research process, rather than just adhering to set criteria after the completion of the study (Guba 1981; Guba and Lincoln 1982; Lincoln and Guba 1985; Morse et al. 2002).

Reliability and validity are two key aspects of all research. Researchers assert that the rigor of qualitative research equates to the concepts of reliability and validity – both are necessary components of quality (Brink 1993; Tappen 2011). However, the precise definition of "quality" has created debate among naturalistic inquirers. Other scholars consider different criteria to describe rigor in qualitative research process (Hall and Rousel 2016). The concepts of reliability and validity have been operationalized eloquently in quantitative texts, but at the same time they were deemed not pertinent to qualitative inquiries in the 1990s. Meticulous attention to the reliability and validity of research studies is particularly vital in qualitative work, where the researcher's subjectivity can so readily cloud the interpretation of the data and where research findings are often questioned or viewed with skepticism by the scientific community (Brink 1993).

There are numerous articles about trustworthiness in the literature that are overly complex, confusing, and full of jargon. Some of these discuss rigor vis-à-vis reliability and validity in a very complicated way. Here, we will first define "rigor," before looking at how "reliability" and "validity" should be applied to qualitative research methods during an inquiry (constructive),

Fundamentals of Qualitative Phenomenological Nursing Research, First Edition. Brigitte S. Cypress.
© 2022 John Wiley & Sons Ltd. Published 2022 by John Wiley & Sons Ltd.

rather than making a post-hoc evaluation. Strategies for attaining reliability and validity will be described, including the criteria and techniques for ensuring their attainment in a study. The discussion will critically focus on the misuse or non-use of the concept of reliability and validity in qualitative inquiries, re-establish their importance, and relate both to the concept of rigor. Reflecting on my own research experience, I will present recommendations for the renewed use of the concept of reliability and validity in qualitative research.

5.1 Rigor versus Trustworthiness

The rigor of qualitative research continues to be challenged even now in the twenty-first century. From the very idea that qualitative research alone is open to questions, it is critical to understand rigor in research. "Rigor" is defined by Merriam-Webster as the quality or state of being very exact, careful, or strictly precise, and by the Oxford English Dictionary as the quality of being thorough and accurate. The term "qualitative rigor" is an oxymoron, as qualitative research is a journey of exploration and discovery that does not lend itself to stiff boundaries (Thomas and Magilvy 2011).

Rigor and truth are always of concern in qualitative research (Houser 2013). Rigor has been used to express attributes related to the qualitative research process (Davies and Dodd 2002; Sandelowski and Barroso 2015). Per Morse et al. (2002), without rigor, research is worthless, becomes fiction, and loses its utility (p. 14). These authors define rigor as the strength of the research design and the appropriateness of the method to answer the questions. It is expected that qualitative studies should be conducted with extreme rigor, because of the potential for subjectivity that is inherent in this type of research. It is more difficult to apply rigor when dealing with narratives and people than with numbers and statistics (Schmidt and Brown 2015). Davies and Dodd (2002) refer rigor to the reliability and validity of research, and aver that inherent to the concept is a quantitative bias. Several researchers argue that reliability and validity pertain to quantitative research, which is unrelated or not pertinent to qualitative inquiry because it is aligned with the positivist view (Rolfe 2006). It is also suggested that a new way of looking at reliability and validity will ensure rigor in qualitative inquiry (Lincoln and Guba 1985; Yin 1994).

From Lincoln and Guba's crucial work in the 1980s, reliability and validity were replaced with the concept of "trustworthiness." Lincoln and Guba (1985) were the first to address rigor in their model of the trustworthiness of qualitative research. Trustworthiness is used as the central concept in their framework to appraise the rigor of a qualitative study. It is defined in different ways by different researchers. It refers to the quality, authenticity, and truthfulness of qualitative research findings. It relates to the degree of trust or confidence readers have in results (Schmidt and Brown 2015, p. 405). Yin (1994) describes trustworthiness as a criterion by which to judge the quality of a research design. Trustworthiness addresses methods that can ensure one has carried out the research process correctly (Guba and Lincoln 1989, p. 245). Manning (1997) considers trustworthiness as a parallel to the empiricist concepts of internal and external validity, reliability, and objectivity. Seale (1999) asserts that trustworthiness is based on the concepts of reliability and validity. Guba and Lincoln (Guba 1981; Guba and Lincoln 1982; Lincoln and Guba 1985) refer to trustworthiness as something that evolved out of four major concerns in research design. Trustworthiness is the goal of a study, and at the same time is something

Table 5.1 The four criteria of trustworthiness: scientific and naturalistic terms.

Criterion	Scientific Term	Naturalistic Term
Truth value	Internal validity	Credibility
Applicability	External validity	Transferability
	Generalizability	
Consistency	Reliability	Dependability
Neutrality	Objectivity	Confirmability

to be judged during a study, after the research has been conducted. The four major traditional criteria are summarized into four questions about truth value, applicability, consistency, and neutrality. From these, Lincoln and Guba (1985) proposed four analogous terms within the naturalistic paradigm: credibility, transferability, dependability, and confirmability. Each of these relates to research activities or steps in which the inquirer should engage in order to be able to safeguard or satisfy each of the criteria and thus attain trustworthiness (Table 5.1). Guba and Lincoln (1982) state:

> The criteria aid inquirers in monitoring themselves and in guiding activities in the field, as a way of determining whether or not various stages in the research are meeting standards for quality and rigor. Finally, the same criteria may be used to render ex-post facto judgments on the products of research, including reports, case studies, or proposed publications. (p. 248)

Standards and checklists were developed in the 1990s based on Lincoln and Guba's (1985) established criteria. However, these standards were thought to cause harm because of confusion over which were appropriate for certain designs and what type of naturalistic inquiry was being undertaken. Thus, researchers interpreted missing data as faults and flaws (Morse 2012). Morse (2012) further claims that the standards became the qualitative researcher's "worst enemies," and that the approach was inappropriate (p. 82). Guba and Lincoln (1989) later proposed a set of guidelines for post-hoc evaluation of a naturalistic inquiry to ensure trustworthiness based on the framework of naturalism and constructivism, beyond the conventional methodological ideas. Aspects of their criteria have been fundamental to the development of standards used to evaluate the quality of qualitative inquiry (Morse et al. 2002).

5.2 The Rigor Debates: Trustworthiness or Reliability and Validity?

A research endeavor, whether quantitative or qualitative, is always evaluated for its worth and merits by peers, experts, reviewers, and readers. Does this mean that a study is differentiated between "good" and "bad"? What determines a "good" from a "bad" inquiry? For a quantitative study, it would mean determining its reliability and validity, and for a qualitative one, its rigor and trustworthiness. According to Golafshani (2003), if the issues of reliability, validity, trustworthiness, and rigor are meant to differentiate "good" from "bad" research, then testing and increasing reliability, validity, trustworthiness, and rigor will be important to the research in any paradigm (p. 602). But, does reliability and validity in quantitative research equate totally to rigor and trustworthiness in qualitative research? There are many ways to assess the "goodness" of a naturalistic inquiry. Guba and Lincoln (1989) ask: "What standards ought apply? . . . goodness criteria like paradigms are rooted in certain assumptions. Thus, it is not appropriate to judge constructivist evaluations by positivistic criteria or standards or vice versa. To each its proper and appropriate set" (p. 251).

Reliability and validity are analogous, and are determined differently than in quantitative inquiry (Morse 2012). The nature and purpose of the quantitative and qualitative traditions are also different, such that it is erroneous to apply the same criteria of worthiness and merit in each case (Agar 1986; Krefting 1991). The qualitative researcher should not focus on quantitatively defined indicators of reliability and validity, but that does not mean that rigorous standards are not appropriate for evaluating findings (Houser 2013). Evaluation, like democracy is a process that, to be at its best, depends upon the application of enlightened and informed self-interest (Guba and Lincoln 1989). Agar (1986), on the other hand, suggests that terms like "reliability" and "validity" are comparative to the quantitative view and do not fit the details of qualitative research (p. 214). A different language is needed to fit the qualitative view. From Leininger (1985), Krefting (1991) asserts that addressing reliability and validity in qualitative research is such a different process that quantitative labels should not be used. The incorrect application of the qualitative criteria of rigor to studies is as problematic as the application of inappropriate quantitative criteria (Krefting 1991). Smith (1989) argues that for qualitative research, this means that the basis of truth or trustworthiness becomes a social agreement. He emphasizes that what is judged true or trustworthy is what we can agree, conditioned by time and place, and is true or trustworthy. Validity standards in qualitative research are even more challenging because of the necessity of incorporating rigor and subjectivity as well as creativity into the scientific process (Johnson 1999). Further, Leininger (1985) claims that it is not whether the data are reliable or valid that is important, but how the terms "reliability" and "validity" are defined. Aside from the debate over whether reliability and validity criteria should be used similarly in qualitative inquiries, there is also the issue of not using the concepts at all in naturalistic studies.

Designing a naturalistic inquiry is very different from the traditional quantitative notion of design, and defining a "good" qualitative inquiry is controversial and has gone through many changes over the years (Morse 2012). First, there is the confusion over the use of terminologies like "rigor" and "trustworthiness." Morse (2015) suggests that it is time to return to return to the terminology of mainstream social science, and to use "rigor" rather than "trustworthiness." Debates also continue about why some qualitative researchers do not use the concepts of reliability and validity in their studies, referring to Lincoln and Guba's (1985) criteria for trustworthiness: transferability, dependability, confirmability and credibility. Morse (2015) further suggests replacing these criteria with *reliability, validity,* and *generalizability.* The importance and centrality of reliability and validity to qualitative inquiries have in some ways been disregarded even in current times. Researchers from the United Kingdom and Europe continue to do so, but not so much those in North America (Morse et al. 2002). According to Morse (2012), this gives the impression that these concepts are of no concern to qualitative research. Morse (1999) asks, "Is the terminology worth making a fuss about?" (p. 717) when Lincoln and Guba (1985) describe trustworthiness, reliability, and validity as analogues. Morse (1999) further articulates that:

> To state that reliability and validity are not pertinent to qualitative inquiry places qualitative research in the realm of being not reliable and not valid. Science is concerned with rigor, and by definition, good rigorous research must be reliable and valid. If qualitative research is unreliable and invalid, then it must not be science. If it is not science, then why should it be funded, published, implemented, or taken seriously? (p. 717)

5.3 Reliability and Validity in Qualitative Research

Reliability and validity should be taken into consideration by qualitative inquirers when designing a study, analyzing results, and judging study quality (Patton 2002), but for too long the criteria used to evaluate rigor have been applied after a research project is completed – a considerably wrong tactic (Morse et al. 2002). Morse et al. (2002) argue that in order for reliability and validity to be actively attained, strategies for ensuring rigor must be built into the qualitative research process per se, not proclaimed only at the end of the inquiry. They suggest that focusing on strategies to establish rigor at the completion of a study (post hoc) rather than during the inquiry exposes investigators to the risk of missing serious threats to reliability and validity until it is too late to correct them. They further assert that the interface between reliability and validity is important, especially for the direction of the analysis process and the development of the study itself.

5.3.1 Reliability

In the social sciences, the whole notion of reliability is problematic in and of itself (Merriam and Leahy 2005). The scientific aspect of reliability assumes that repeated measures of a phenomenon (with the same results) using objective methods establish the truth of findings (Black and Champion 1976; Hammersley 1987; Johnston and Pennypacker 1980; Lehner 1979). Merriam (1998) states that "The more times the findings of a study can be replicated, the more stable or reliable the phenomenon is thought to be" (p. 55). In other words, reliability is based on the idea of replicability (Golafshani 2003; Johnston and Pennypacker 1980; Winter 2000), repeatability (Campbell and Fisk 1959; Golafshani 2003; Kerlinger 1964; Merriam 1998; Merriam and Leahy 2005; Morse 2012; Patton 2002; Smith 1989; Winter 2000), and stability (Kerlinger 1964; Leininger 1985;

Table 5.2 Terms related to reliability.

Term	Authors
Repeatability	Black and Champion (1976), Campbell and Fisk (1959), Golafshani (2003), Hammersley (1987), Johnston and Pennypacker (1980), Lehner (1979), Morse (1991), Winter (2000)
Replicability	Golafshani (2003), Merriam (1998), Winter (2000)
Consistency	Clont (1992), Guba and Lincoln (1989), Kerlinger (1964), Lincoln and Guba (1985), Morse (1991), Seale (1999)
Stability	Johnston and Pennypacker (1980), Kerlinger (1964), Lehner (1979), Morse (1991)

Simco and Warin 1997) in results and observations. The issue are that human behaviors and interactions are never static or the same, and measurements and observations can be repeatedly wrong. Further, researchers have argued that the concept of reliability is misleading and has no relevance in qualitative research related to the notion of "measurement method" as in quantitative studies (Morse 1991; Winter 2000). It is a fact that quantitative research is supported by the positivist or scientific paradigm that regards the world as made up of observable, measurable facts. Qualitative research, on the other hand, produces findings not arrived at by means of statistical procedures or other means of quantification. Based on the constructivist paradigm, it is a naturalistic inquiry that seeks to understand phenomena in context-specific settings in which the researcher does not attempt to manipulate the phenomenon of interest (Krefting 1991). If reliability is used as a criterion in qualitative research, it will show that the study is "not good." A thorough description of the entire research process that allows for inter-subjectivity is what indicates good quality when using qualitative methodology. Reliability is based on consistency and care in the application of research practices, which are reflected in the visibility of research practices, analysis, and conclusions, in an open account that remains mindful of the partiality and limits of the research findings (Davies and Dodd 2002). The terms related to reliability are presented in Table 5.2.

5.3.2 Validity

Validity is broadly defined by Merriam-Webster as the state of being well grounded or justifiable, relevant, meaningful, logical, confirming to accepted principles, or being sound, just, and well-founded. The issues surrounding the use and nature of the term "validity" in qualitative research are controversial and many. It is a highly debated topic in both social and educational research, and is still often the subject of debate (Creswell 2007). The traditional criteria for validity find their roots in a positivist tradition, and to an extent positivism has been defined by a systematic theory of validity (Golafshani 2003). Validity is rooted in empirical conceptions as universal laws, evidence, objectivity, truth, actuality, deduction, reason, fact, and mathematical data, among many other things. Validity in research is concerned with the accuracy and truthfulness of scientific findings (van Manen 1990). A valid study should demonstrate what actually exists and be accurate, and a valid instrument or measure should actually measure what it is supposed to measure (Brink 1993; Golafshani 2003; Le Compte and Goetz 1982; Merriam and Leahy 2005; Morse 1991, 1999).

Novice researchers can become easily perplexed in attempting to understand the notion of validity in qualitative inquiry (van Manen 1990). There are a multitude of similar terms in the literature, such as "authenticity," "goodness," "adequacy," "trustworthiness," "verisimilitude," "credibility," and "plausibility" (Altheide and Johnson 1994; Creswell and Miller 2000; Hammersley 1990; Lather 1993; Le Compte and Goetz 1982; Lincoln and Guba 1985; Lub 2015). Validity is not a single, fixed, or universal concept, but rather a contingent construct, inescapably grounded in the processes and intentions of particular research methodologies (Kerlinger 1964). Some qualitative researchers have argued that the term "validity" is not applicable to qualitative research and have related it to terms such as "quality," "rigor," and "trustworthiness" (Campbell and Fisk 1959; Davies and Dodd 2002; Golafshani 2003; Lincoln and Guba 1985; Maxwell 1992, 1996; Morse 1991; Stenbacka 2001). I argue that the concepts of reliability and validity are overarching constructs that can be appropriately used in both quantitative and qualitative methodologies. To validate means to investigate, to question, and to theorize – all of which are activities aimed at ensuring rigor in a qualitative inquiry. For Leininger (1985), the term "validity" in a qualitative sense means gaining knowledge and understanding of the nature (i.e., the meaning, attributes, and characteristics) of the phenomenon under study. A qualitative method seeks for a certain quality that is typical for the phenomenon or that makes the phenomenon different than others.

Some naturalistic inquirers agree that assuring validity is a process whereby ideals are sought through attention to specified criteria and appropriate techniques are employed to address any threats to the validity of a naturalistic inquiry. However, other researchers argue that procedures and techniques are not an assurance of validity and will not necessarily produce sound data or credible conclusions (Campbell and Fisk 1959; Creswell and Miller 2000; Merriam 1998). Thus, some argue that we should abandon the concept of validity and seek alternative criteria with which to judge our work. *Criteria* are the standards or rule to be upheld as ideals in qualitative research on which a judgment or decision may be based (Morse et al. 2002; Sandelowski 1993), whereas *techniques* are the methods employed to diminish identified validity threats (Schwandt 1996). Criteria for some researchers are things used to test the quality of the research design, while for others they are the goal of the study. There is also a trend toward treating standards, goals, and criteria synonymously. I concur with Morse (1999) that introducing parallel terminology and criteria diminishes qualitative inquiry relative to mainstream science and scientific legitimacy. The development of alternative criteria compromises the issue of rigor. We must work to have a consensus toward criteria and terminology that are used in mainstream science and their attainment during the research process rather than at the end of a qualitative study.

Despite all these issues, researchers have developed a number of validity criteria and techniques over the years, as summarized in Table 5.3. The techniques for demonstrating validity are presented in Table 5.4.

Table 5.3 Synthesis of validity criteria development.

Authors	Validity Criteria
Lincoln and Guba (1985)	
Guba and Lincoln (1989)	Truth value, applicability, consistency, neutrality
Sandelowski (1993)	Credibility, fittingness, auditability, confirmability, creativity, artfulness
Marshall (1990)	Goodness, canons of evidence
Smith (1990)	Moral and ethical component
Eisenhart and Howe (1992)	Completeness, appropriateness, comprehensiveness, credibility, significance
Maxwell (1992, 1996)	Descriptive validity, interpretive validity, theoretical validity, evaluative validity, generalizability
Altheide and Johnson (1994)	Plausibility, relevance, credibility, importance of topic
Leininger (1994)	Credibility, confirmability, meaning in context, recurrent patterning, saturation, transferability
Morse (1991)	Credibility, confirmability, meaning-in-context, recurrent patterning, saturation and transferability
Lincoln (1995)	Positionality, community as arbiter, voice, critical subjectivity, reciprocity, sacredness, sharing perquisites of privilege
Merriam (1998)	Internal validity: triangulation, member checks, peer examination, statement of researcher's biases, assumptions-presenting the orientation, submersion/engagement in the research situation
	External validity: thick description, multisite design, modal comparison, sampling within
Thorne (1997)	Methodological integrity, representative credibility, analytic logic, interpretive authority
Popay et al. (1998)	Interpretation of subjective meaning, description of social context and flexibility of design, attention to lay knowledge: theoretical basis, sampling strategy, scope of data collection, description of data collected, concern with generalizability and typicality
Healy and Perry (2000)	Triangulation of several data sources and their interpretations with those multiple perceptions in the realism paradigm
Creswell and Miller (2000)	Constructivist paradigm/lens:
	Researcher: disconfirming evidence
	Study participants: prolonged engagement in the field
	External reviewers/readers: thick, rich description
Whittemore et al. (2001)	Primary criteria: credibility, authenticity criticality, and integrity;
	Secondary criteria: explicitness, vividness, creativity, thoroughness, congruence, and sensitivity

Table 5.3 (Continued)

Authors	Validity Criteria
Davies and Dodd (2002)	Investigator's attentiveness, empathy, carefulness, sensitivity, respect, honesty, reflection, conscientiousness, engagement, awareness, openness, context
Morse et al. (2002)	Investigator responsiveness: researcher's creativity, sensitivity, flexibility and skill in using the verification strategies that determines the reliability and validity of the evolving study
	Verification strategies: methodological coherence, sample must be appropriate and adequate, collecting and analyzing data concurrently, saturation thinking theoretically, theory development

Source: Whittemore, R., Chase, S. K., & Mandle, C. L. (2001). Validity in qualitative research. *Qualitative Health Research*, 11(2): 117–132.

Table 5.4 Techniques for demonstrating validity.

Technique	Methods
Design consideration	Developing a self-conscious research design
	Sampling decisions (i.e., sampling adequacy)
	Employing triangulation
	Giving voice
Data generation	Articulating data collection decisions
	Demonstrating prolonged engagement
	Demonstrating persistent observation
	Providing verbatim transcription
	Demonstrating saturation
Analytical procedures	Articulating data analysis decisions
	Member checking
	Expert checking
	Drawing data reduction tables
	Exploring rival explanations
	Performing a literature review
	Analyzing negative case analysis
	Memoing
	Reflexive journaling
	Bracketing
Presentation	Providing an audit trail
	Providing evidence that support interpretations
	Acknowledging the researcher's perspective
	Providing thick descriptions

Source: Whittemore, R., Chase, S. K., & Mandle, C. L. (2001). Validity in qualitative research. *Qualitative Health Research*, 11(2): 117–132.

5.4 Exemplar: Reliability and Validity as Means of Ensuring the Quality of Findings in a Phenomenological Study in the ICU

Reliability and validity are two factors that any qualitative researcher should be concerned about while designing a study, analyzing results, and judging study quality. Just as the quantitative investigator must attend to the question of how external and internal validity, reliability, and objectivity will be provided for in their design, so must the naturalistic inquirer consider credibility, transferability, dependability, and confirmability (Lincoln and Guba 1985, p. 247). Lincoln and Guba (1985) clearly established these four criteria as benchmarks for quality based on the identification of four aspects of trustworthiness that are relevant to both quantitative and qualitative studies: truth value, applicability, consistency, and neutrality. Guba (1981) states: "It is to these concerns that the criteria must speak" (p. 79).

The rigor of a naturalistic form of inquiry such as phenomenology may be operationalized using the criteria of credibility, transferability, dependability, and confirmability. In my exemplar phenomenological study, I aimed to understand and illuminate the meaning of the phenomenon of the lived experiences of patients, their family members, and their nurses during critical illness in the intensive care unit (ICU). From Lincoln and Guba (1985), I first asked: "How can I persuade my audience that the research findings of my inquiry are worth paying attention to, and worth taking account of?" My answers were based on the identified four criteria set forth by Lincoln and Guba (1985).

Credibility – the accurate and truthful depiction of a participant's lived experience – was achieved through *prolonged engagement* and *persistent observation* to learn the context of the phenomenon in which it was embedded and to minimize distortions that might creep into the data. To achieve this, I spent six months with nurses, patients, and their families in the ICU to become oriented to the situation and to build trust and rapport with the participants. *Peer debriefing* was done through meetings and discussions with an expert qualitative researcher to allow for questions and critiques of field journals and research activities. *Triangulation* was achieved by cross-checking the data and having two qualitative researchers make interpretations within and across each category of participants. *Member checks* were accomplished by constantly checking the data and making interpretations with the participants from whom the data were solicited.

Transferability was enhanced by using the *purposive sampling method* and providing *a thick description and a robust data set* with a wide possible range of information through the detailed and accurate descriptions of the patients', family members', and nurses' lived ICU experiences, and by continuously returning to the texts. In this study, recruitment of participants and data collection continued until the data were redundant, consistently repeated/replicated, and complete. According to Morse et al. (2002), interviewing additional participants is done in order to increase the scope, adequacy, and appropriateness of the data. I immersed myself into the phenomenon in order to know, describe, and understand it fully, comprehensively, and thoroughly. Special care was given to the collection, identification, and analysis of all data pertinent to the study.

The audio-taped data were meticulously transcribed by a professional transcriber for future scrutiny. During the analysis phase, every attempt was made to document all aspects of the analysis. Analysis in qualitative research refers to the categorization and ordering of information in such a way as to make sense of it and to provide a final report that is true and accurate (Merriam 1998). Every effort was made to coordinate methodological and analytical material. After I categorized and was able to make sense of the transcribed data, I made all efforts to illuminate themes and descriptors as they emerged.

Lincoln and Guba (1985) describe "dependability" in qualitative research, which closely corresponds to the notion of "reliability" in quantitative research. Dependability was achieved by having two expert qualitative nursing researchers review the transcribed material to validate the themes and descriptors identified. In order to validate my findings related to the themes, a doctoral-prepared nursing colleague was asked to review some of the transcribed material. Any new themes and descriptors illuminated by my colleague were acknowledged and considered, and then compared to my own thematic analysis from the whole of the participants' transcribed data. If the theme identified by the colleague did not appear in my own thematic analysis, it was agreed by both analysts not to use it. It was my goal that both analysts should agree on the findings related to themes and meanings within the transcribed material.

Confirmability was met by maintaining a *reflexive Journal* during the research process in order to keep notes and document daily introspections that might be beneficial and pertinent during the study. An *audit trail* was conducted to examine the processes whereby data were collected, analyzed, and interpreted. This trail took the form of documentation (the actual interview notes taken) and a running account of the process (my daily field journal). I maintained self-awareness of my role as the sole instrument of this study. After each interview, I retired in a private room to document additional perceptions and recollections from the interviews. The rigor criteria applied to the exemplar phenomenological study are presented in Table 5.5.

Through reflexivity and bracketing, I was always on guard against my own biases, assumptions, beliefs, and presuppositions, with the awareness that complete reduction is not possible. Van Manen (1990) states: "If we simply try to forget or ignore what we already know, we may find that the presuppositions persistently creep back into our reflections" (p. 47). During data collection and analysis, I made my orientation and

Table 5.5 Trustworthiness criteria applied to the exemplar phenomenological study.

Criterion	Methods
Credibility	Prolonged engagement, persistent observation, peer debriefing, triangulation, member checking
Transferability	Purposive sampling, thick description and robust data
Dependability	Use of overlap methods (kind of triangulation), same methods as in credibility
Confirmability	Audit trail, reflexive journaling

pre-understanding of critical illness and critical care explicit, but held them deliberately at bay and bracketed them. Aside from Lincoln and Guba's (1985) four criteria for rigor, a question arises as to the reliability of the researcher as the sole instrument of a study.

Reliability related to the researcher as the sole instrument of data collection and analysis is a limitation of any phenomenological study. The use of humans as instruments is not a new concept. Lincoln and Guba (1985) articulate that humans uniquely qualify as the instrument of choice for naturalistic inquiry. Some of the giants of conventional inquiry have recognized that humans can provide data very nearly as reliable as that produced by "more" objective means. These are formidable characteristics, but they are meaningless if the human instrument is not also trustworthy. However, no human instrument is expected to be perfect. Humans have flaws and can commit errors. When Lincoln and Guba (1985) assert that qualitative methods come more easily to hand when the instrument is a human being, they mean that the human as instrument is inclined toward methods that are extensions of normal activities. They believe that the human will tend, therefore, toward interviewing, observing, mining available documents and records, taking account of non-verbal cues, and interpreting inadvertent unobtrusive measures, all of which are complex tasks. Also, one would not expect an individual to function adequately as a human instrument without an extensive background or extensive training and experience.

This exemplar study has reliability in that I have acquired knowledge and the required training for research at a doctoral level with the professional and expert guidance of a mentor. As Lincoln and Guba (1985) state: "Performance can be improved . . . when that learning is guided by an experienced mentor, remarkable improvements in human instrumental performance can be achieved" (p. 195). While reliability in quantitative research depends on instrument construction, in qualitative research the researcher is the sole instrument of the study. Reliable research is credible research. Credibility of qualitative research depends on the ability and effort of the researcher (Golafshani 2003). We have established that a study can be reliable without being valid but cannot be valid without being reliable.

Establishing validity is a major challenge when a qualitative research project uses a single cross-sectional unstructured interview as the basis for data collection. How can one make judgments about the validity of the data? In qualitative research, the validity of the findings is related to the careful recording and continual verification of the data that the researcher gathers during the investigative practice. If the validity or trustworthiness can be maximized or tested, then more credible and defensible results may lead to generalizability as the structure for both doing and documenting high-quality qualitative research. Therefore, the quality of a research project is related to the generalizability of the results, and thereby to the testing and validity or rigor of the research.

One potential threat to validity that researchers need to consider is researcher bias. This is frequently an issue because qualitative research is open and comparatively less structured than quantitative research. That is because qualitative research tends to be exploratory. Researcher bias results most often from selective observation and selective recording of information, and from allowing one's personal views and perspectives to affect how data are interpreted and how the research is conducted. Therefore, it is very important that researchers are aware of their own perceptions and opinions, because these may taint their findings and conclusions. I brought all my past experiences and knowledge into the study, but learned to set aside my own strongly held perceptions, preconceptions, and opinions. I truly listened to the participants in order to learn their stories, experiences, and meanings.

The key strategy used to understand researcher bias is called *reflexivity*. Reflexivity means that the researcher actively engages in critical self-reflection about the potential biases and predispositions that they bring to the qualitative study. Through reflexivity, researchers become more self-aware, and can monitor and attempt to control their biases. Phenomenological researchers can recognize that their interpretation is correct because the reflective process awakens in them an inner moral impulse (Morse et al. 2002; Sparkes 2001). I did my best to be always on guard against my own biases, preconceptions, and assumptions.

Husserl (1931) made some key conceptual elaborations that led him to assert that an attempt to hold in suspension prior beliefs about a phenomenon under study in order to perceive it more clearly is necessary in phenomenological research. This technique is called *bracketing*. Bracketing is another strategy used to control bias. Husserl (1931) explained further that phenomenological reduction is the process of defining the pure essence of a psychological phenomenon. Phenomenological reduction is a process whereby empirical subjectivity is suspended so that pure consciousness may be defined in its essential and absolute *being*. This is accomplished by a method of bracketing empirical data away from consideration. Bracketing leaves pure consciousness, pure phenomena, and the pure ego as the residue of phenomenological reduction. Husserl (1931) used the term *epoche* (Greek for "a cessation") to refer to this suspension of judgment regarding the true nature of reality. Bracketed judgment is an *epoche* or suspension of inquiry, which places in brackets whatever facts belong to essential *being*.

I carried out bracketing to separate my assumptions and biases from the essences of the data, and therefore to achieve an understanding of the phenomenon as experienced by the participants of the study. I presented the collected and analyzed data to the participants and asked them whether the narrative was accurate and a true reflection of their experiences. I further presented my interpretation and descriptions of the narratives to the participants to achieve credibility. They were given the opportunity to review the transcripts and to modify them if they wished to do so. As I was the sole instrument in obtaining data for this phenomenological study, I aimed that the participants should be able to perceive their experiences as lived. As qualitative research designs are flexible and emergent in nature, there will always be study limitations.

Awareness of the limitations of a research study is crucial for researchers. One limitation of this exemplar phenomenological study as a naturalistic inquiry was my inability to fully design and provide specific ideas necessary for the study before it started. According to Lincoln and Guba (1985), naturalistic studies are virtually impossible to design in any definitive way before they are actually undertaken:

> Designing a naturalistic study means something very different from the traditional notion of "design" – which as often as not meant the specification of a statistical design with its attendant field conditions and controls. Most of the requirements normally laid down for a design statement cannot be met by naturalists because the naturalistic inquiry is largely emergent. (p. 248)

Within the naturalistic paradigm, designs must be emergent rather than pre-ordinate because: (i) meaning is determined by context to such a great extent – for this phenomenological study, the phenomenon and context were the experience of critical illness in the ICU; (ii) the existence of multiple realities constrains the development of a design based on only one (the investigator's) construction; (iii) what will be learned at a site is always dependent on the interaction between the investigator and the context, and the interaction is not fully predictable; and (iv) the nature of mutual shapings cannot be known until they are witnessed. These factors underscore the indeterminacy under which naturalistic inquiry functions. The design must therefore be "played by ear": it must unfold, cascade, and emerge. It does not follow, however, that because not all of the elements of the design can be pre-specified in a naturalistic inquiry, none of them can. Design in the naturalistic sense means planning for certain broad contingencies without indicating exactly what will be done in relation to each (Lincoln and Guba 1985).

5.5 The Rigor Debate Continues: How Do We Move Forward?

Reliability and validity are fundamental concepts that should be continually operationalized to meet the conditions of a qualitative inquiry. Morse (1999) articulates that "By refusing to acknowledge the centrality of reliability and validity in qualitative methods, qualitative methodologists have inadvertently fostered the default notion that qualitative research must therefore be unreliable and invalid, lacking in rigor, and unscientific" (p. 15). Sparkes (2001) asserts that Morse (1999) is right in warning us that turning our backs on such fundamental concepts as validity could cost us dearly. This affects how we mentor novices, early career researchers, and doctoral students in their qualitative research works.

Reliability is inherently integrated and internally necessary in order to attain validity (Lincoln and Guba 1985; Smith 1989). I concur with the use of the term "rigor" rather than "trustworthiness" in naturalistic studies. I have also discussed how I accede that strategies for ensuring rigor must be built into the qualitative research process per se rather than evaluated only after an inquiry is conducted. Threats to reliability and validity cannot be actively addressed by using standards and criteria applied at the end of a study. Rigor must be upheld by the researcher during the investigation rather the external judges of the completed study. Whether a study is quantitative or qualitative, rigor is a desired goal that is met through the inclusion of different philosophical perspectives inherent in a qualitative inquiry and the strategies that are specific to each methodological approach, including the verification techniques to be observed during the research process. It also involves the researcher's creativity, sensitivity, flexibility, and skill in using the verification strategies that determine the reliability and validity of the evolving study.

Lincoln and Guba's (1985) standards of validity demonstrate the necessity and convenience of overarching principles to all qualitative research, yet there is a need for a re-conceptualization of criteria of validity in qualitative research. The development of validity criteria in qualitative research poses theoretical issues, not simply technical ones (Mishler 2000). Whittemore et al. (2001) explored the historical development of validity criteria in qualitative research and synthesized findings reflecting a contemporary re-conceptualization of the debate and dialogue in the literature over the years. They further presented primary (credibility, authenticity, criticality, and integrity) and secondary (explicitness, vividness, creativity, thoroughness, congruence, and sensitivity) validity criteria to be used in the evaluative process (Whittemore et al. 2001). Prior to the work of Whittemore and colleagues, Creswell and Miller (2000) asserted that the constructivist lens and paradigm choice should guide validity evaluation and procedures from the perspectives of the researcher (disconfirming evidence), the study participants (prolonged engagement in the field), and external reviewers/readers (thick, rich description). Morse et al. (2002) presented six major evaluation criteria for validity and asserted that they were congruent and appropriate within the philosophy of the qualitative tradition. These six criteria are credibility, confirmability, meaning-in-context, recurrent patterning, saturation, and transferability. The synthesis of validity criteria is presented in Table 5.3.

Common validity techniques in qualitative research refer to design consideration, data generation, analytic procedures, and presentation (Schwandt 1996). Design consideration involves development of a self-conscious design, paradigm assumption, the purposeful choice of a small sample of informants relevant to the study, and the use of an inductive approach. A purposive sampling enhances the transferability of the results. Interpretivist and constructivist inquiry follows an inductive approach that is flexible and emergent in design, with some uncertainty and fluidity within the context of the phenomenon of interest (Moskal et al. 2002; Schwandt 1996), and not based on a set of determinate rules (Smith 1990). The researcher does not work with a priori theories; rather, these are expected to emerge from the inquiry. Data are analyzed inductively from specific, raw units of information in order to define questions that can be followed up (Lincoln and Guba 1985). Qualitative studies also follow a naturalistic and constructivist paradigm. Creswell and Miller (2000) suggest that validity is affected by the researchers' perceptions of validity, and by their choice of paradigm assumption. Determining fit of paradigm to focus is an essential aspect of a naturalistic inquiry (Lincoln and Guba 1985). Paradigms rest upon sets of beliefs called axioms (Lincoln and Guba 1985). Based on naturalistic axioms, the researchers should ask questions related to multiplicity or complex constructions of the phenomenon, the degree of investigator–phenomenon interaction, the indeterminacy that will be introduced into the study, and the degree of context dependence if values are likely to be crucial to the outcome, and the constraints that may be placed on the researcher by a variety of significant others (Lincoln and Guba 1985).

Validity during data generation is evaluated through the researcher's ability to articulate data collection decisions, demonstrate prolonged engagement, engage in persistent observation, provide verbatim transcription, and achieve data repeatability and redundancy (Schwandt 1996). Methods are means of collecting evidence to support validity, including obtaining data by considering the context for a purpose. The human instrument operating in an indeterminate situation falls back on techniques such as interview, observation, unobtrusive measures, documentation, record analysis, and non-verbal cues (Lincoln and Guba 1985). Some authors note that rejecting methods or technical procedures as an assurance of the validity of a qualitative study will depend upon the skills and sensitivities of the researcher, and how they see themselves as knowers and inquirers (Phillips 1987; Whittemore et al. 2001). The understanding of a phenomenon is valid if the participants are given the opportunity to speak freely according to their own knowledge structures and perceptions. Validity is therefore achieved when using the method of open-ended, unstructured interviews with strategically chosen participants (Morse 1991). We also know that a thorough description of the entire research process enabling unconditional inter-subjectivity is what indicates good quality when using the qualitative method. This enhances a clearer and better analysis of data.

Analytical procedures are vital in qualitative research (Schwandt 1996). Not very much can be said about data analysis in advance of a qualitative study (Lincoln and Guba 1985). Data analysis is not an inclusive phase that can be marked out as occurring at some singular time during the inquiry (Lincoln and Guba 1985). It begins from the very first data collection, in order to facilitate emergent design and grounding of theory. Validity in a study is thus represented by the truthfulness of the findings after a careful analysis (Schwandt 1996). Consequently, qualitative researchers seek to illuminate and extrapolate findings to similar situations (Golafshani 2003; Mishler 1990). It is a fact, however, that the interpretations of any given social phenomenon may reflect, in part, the biases and prejudices the interpreters bring to the task, and the criteria and logic they follow in completing it (Reason 1991). In any case, individuals will draw different conclusions on the debate surrounding validity, and will make different judgments as a result (Altheide and Johnson 1994). There are a wide array of analytic techniques that the qualitative researcher can choose from, based on the contextual factors that will help contribute to the decision as to which technique will optimally reflect specific criteria of validity. Presentation of findings is accomplished by providing an audit trail and evidence that supports interpretations, acknowledging the researcher's perspective, and providing thick descriptions. Morse et al. (2002) set forth strategies for ensuring validity that include investigator responsiveness and verification through methodological coherence, theoretical sampling, sampling adequacy, an active analytic stance, and data redundancy. They state that "These strategies, when used appropriately, force the researcher to correct both the direction of the analysis and the development of the study as necessary, thus ensuring reliability and validity of the completed project" (p. 17). Recently, Morse (2015) presented the strategies for ensuring validity in a qualitative study: prolonged engagement, persistent observation, thick and rich description, negative case analysis, peer-review or debriefing, clarifying researcher's bias, member checking, external audits, and triangulation. These strategies can be upheld with the help of an expert mentor, who in turn can guide and affect the reliability and validity of early-career researchers' and doctoral students' qualitative research works. Techniques for demonstrating validity are summarized in Table 5.4.

Qualitative researchers and students alike must be pro-active in and take responsibility for ensuring the rigor of a research study. A lot of times, rigor takes the backseat in new researchers' work due to their novice abilities, lack of proper mentorship, and issues with time and funding. Students should conduct projects that are small in scope, guided by an expert naturalistic inquirer, in order to come up with a product with depth and gain the grounding experience necessary to become an excellent researcher. Attending to rigor throughout the research process will have important ramifications for qualitative inquiry (Morse et al. 2002; Smith 1989).

Qualitative research is not intended to be scary or beyond the grasp of novices and doctoral students. Conducting a naturalistic inquiry is a process of exploration, discovery, description, and understanding that transcends one's own research journey. Attending to the rigor of qualitative research is a vital part of the investigative process that offers critique and thus further development of the science.

5.6 Conclusion

This chapter presented the concept of rigor in qualitative research using a phenomenological study as an exemplar. It provided a synthesis of the historical development of validity criteria over the years, including the re-conceptualization and renewed use of the concepts of reliability and validity in qualitative research. The insights provided will help novice phenomenological researchers have a better background in and conceptual grasp of the complexity of rigor in qualitative inquiries, and thus apply them in their own research journeys.

References

Agar, M. (1986). Speaking of Ethnography. Sage Publications.

Altheide, D.L. and Johnson, J.M. (1994). Criteria for Assessing Interpretive Validity in Qualitative Research. Sage Publications.

Black, J.A. and Champion, D.J. (1976). Methods and Issues in Social Research. Wiley.

Brink, H.I. (1993). Validity and reliability in qualitative research. Curationis 16 (2): 35–38.

Campbell, D.T. and Fisk, D.W. (1959). Convergent and discriminant validation by the multitrait multimethod matrix. Psychological Bulleting 56 (2): 81–106.

Creswell, J.W. (2007). Qualitative Inquiry and Research Design: Choosing Among Five Approaches, 2e. Sage Publications.

Creswell, J.W. and Miller, D.L. (2000). Determining validity in qualitative inquiry. Theory into Practice 39 (3): 124–131.

Davies, D. and Dodd, J. (2002). Qualitative research and the question of rigor. Qualitative Health Research 12 (2): 279–289.

Eisenhart, M.A. and Howe, K.R. (1992). Validity in educational research. In: The Handbook of Qualitative Research in Education (eds. M.D. LeCompte, W.L. Millroy and J. Preissle), 643–680. Academic Press.

Golafshani, N. (2003). Understanding reliability and validity in qualitative research. The Qualitative Report 8 (4): 597–607.

Guba, E.G. (1981). Criteria for assessing the trustworthiness of naturalistic inquiries. Education Communication and Technology Journal 29: 75–91.

Guba, E.G. and Lincoln, Y.S. (1982). Epistemological and methodological bases of naturalistic inquiry. Education Communication and Technology Journal 30: 233–252.

Guba, E.G. and Lincoln, Y.S. (1989). Fourth Generation Evaluation. Sage Publications.

Hall, H.R. and Rousel, L.A. (2016). Evidence-Based Practice: An Integrative Approach to Research, Administration and Practice, 2e. Jones and Bartlett Learning.

Hammersley, M. (1987). Some notes on the terms "validity" and "reliability". British Educational Research Journal 13 (1): 73–82.

Hammersley, M. (1990). Reading Ethnographic Research: A Critical Guide. Longmans.

Healy, M. and Perry, C. (2000). Comprehensive criteria to judge validity and reliability of qualitative research within the realism paradigm. Qualitative Market Research 3 (3): 118–126.

Houser, J. (2013). Nursing Research: Reading, Using, and Creating Evidence, 2e. Jones and Bartlett Learning.

Husserl, E. (1931). Ideas: General Introduction to Pure Phenomenology (trans. W.R.B. Gibson). Macmillan.

Johnson, M. (1999). Observations on positivism and pseudoscience in qualitative nursing research. Journal of Advanced Nursing 30 (1): 67–73.

Johnston, J.M. and Pennypacker, H.S. (1980). Strategies and Tactics of Human Behavioural Research. Lawrence Erlbaum Associates.

Kerlinger, F. (1964). Foundations of Behavioural Research. Holt.

Krefting, L. (1991). Rigor in qualitative research: the assessment of trustworthiness. American Journal of Occupational Therapy 45: 214–222.

Lather, P. (1993). Fertile obsession: validity after poststructuralism. The Sociological Quarterly 34 (4): 673–693.

Le Compte, M.D. and Goetz, J.P. (1982). Problems of reliability and validity in ethnographic research. Review of Educational Research 52 (1): 31–60.

Lehner, P.N. (1979). Handbook of Ethological Methods. STPM Press.

Leininger, M.M. (1985). Nature, rationale and importance of qualitative research methods in nursing. In: Qualitative Research Methods in Nursing (ed. M.M. Leininger), 1–28. Grune & Stratton.

Leininger, M.M. (1994). Evaluation criteria and critique of qualitative research studies. In: Critical Issues in Qualitative Research Methods, 1e (ed. J.M. Morse), 95–115. Sage Publications.

Lincoln, Y.S. (1995). Emerging criteria for quality in qualitative and interpretive research. Qualitative Inquiry 3: 275–289.

Lincoln, Y.S. and Guba, E.G. (1985). Naturalistic Inquiry. Sage Publications.

Lub, V. (2015). Validity in qualitative evaluation: linking purposes, paradigms, and perspectives. International Journal of Qualitative Methods 14: 1–8.

van Manen, M. (1990). Researching Lived Experience: Human Science for an Action Sensitive Pedagogy. State University of New York Press.

Manning, K. (1997). Authenticity in constructivist inquiry: methodological considerations without prescription. Qualitative Inquiry 3 (1): 93–115.

Marshall, C. (1990). Goodness criteria: Are they objective or judgement calls? In: The Paradigm Dialog (ed. E.G. Guba), 188–197. Sage Publications.

Maxwell, J.A. (1992). Understanding and validity in qualitative research. Harvard Educational Review 62 (3): 279–299.

Maxwell, J.A. (1996). Qualitative Research Design: An Interactive Approach. Sage Publications.

Merriam, S.B. (1998). Qualitative Research and Case Study Applications in Education. Jossey-Bass.

Merriam, S.B. and Leahy, B. (2005). Learning transfer: a review of the research in adult education and training. PAACE Journal of Lifelong Learning 14: 1–24.

Mishler, E.G. (1990). Validation in inquiry-guided research: the role of exemplars in narrative studies. Harvard Educational Review 60 (4): 415–442.

Mishler, E.G. (2000). Validation in inquiry-guided research: the role of exemplars in narrative studies. In: Acts of Inquiry in Qualitative Research (eds. B.M. Brizuela, J.P. Stewart, R.G. Carrillo and J.G. Berger), 119–146. Harvard Educational Review.

Morse, J. (1991). Qualitative nursing research: a free for all? In: Qualitative Nursing Research: A Contemporary Dialogue, 2e (ed. J. Morse), 14–22. Sage Publications.

Morse, J.M. (1999). Myth #93: reliability and validity are not relevant to qualitative inquiry. Qualitative Health Research 9 (6): 717.

Morse, J. (2012). Qualitative Health Research: Creating a New Discipline, 1e. Routledge.

Morse, J. (2015). Critical analysis of strategies for determining rigor in qualitative inquiry. Qualitative Health Research 25 (9): 1212–1222.

Morse, J.M., Barrett, M., Mayan, M. et al. (2002). Verification strategies for establishing reliability and validity in qualitative research. International Journal of Qualitative Methods 1 (2): 13–22.

Moskal, B., Leydens, J., and Pavelich, M. (2002). Validity, reliability and the assessment of engineering education. Journal of Engineering Education 91 (3): 351–354.

Patton, M.Q. (2002). Qualitative Evaluation and Research Methods, 3e. Sage Publications.

Phillips, D.C. (1987). Validity in qualitative research: why the worry about warrant will not wane. Education and Urban Society 20 (1): 9–24.

Popay, J., Rogers, A., and Williams, G. (1998). Rationale and standards for the systematic review of qualitative literature in health services research. Qualitative Health Research 8: 341–351.

Reason, P. (1991). Issues of validity in new paradigm research. In: Human Inquiry (eds. P. Reason and J. Rowan), 239–250. Wiley.

Rolfe, G. (2006). Validity, trustworthiness and rigour: quality and the idea of qualitative research. Journal of Advance Nursing 53 (3): 304–310.

Sandelowski, M. (1993). Rigor or rigor mortis: the problem of rigor in qualitative research revisited. Advances in Nursing Science 16 (2): 1–8.

Sandelowski, M. and Barroso, J. (2015). Reading qualitative studies. International Journal of Qualitative Methods 1 (1): 74–108.

Schmidt, N.A. and Brown, J. (2015). Evidence-Based Practice for Nurses: Appraisal and Application of Research, 3e. Jones and Bartlett.

Schwandt, T.A. (1996). Farewell to criteriology. Qualitative Inquiry 2 (1): 58–72.

Seale, C. (1999). Quality in qualitative research. Qualitative Inquiry 5 (4): 465–478.

Simco, N. and Warin, J. (1997). Validity in image-based research: an elaborated illustration of the issues. British Educational Research Association Journal 23 (5): 661–673.

Smith, J. (1989). The Nature of Social and Educational Inquiry: Empiricism Versus Interpretation. Ablex.

Smith, J.K. (1990). Alternative research paradigms and the problem of criteria. In: The Paradigm Dialog (ed. E.G. Guba), 167–187. Sage Publications.

Sparkes, A. (2001). Myth 94: qualitative researchers will agree about validity. Qualitative Health Research 11 (4): 538–555.

Stenbacka, C. (2001). Qualitative research requires quality concepts of its own. Manage Decision 39 (7): 551–555.

Tappen, R.M. (2011). Advanced Nursing Research: From Theory to Practice. Jones & Bartlett Learning.

Thomas, E. and Magilvy, J.K. (2011). Qualitative rigor or research validity in qualitative research. Journal for Specialist in Pediatric Nursing 16 (2): 151–155.

Thorne, S. (1997). The art (and science) of critiquing qualitative research. In: Completing a Qualitative Project: Details and Dialogue (ed. J.M. Morse), 117–132. Sage Publications.

Whittemore, R., Chase, S.K., and Mandle, C.L. (2001). Validity in qualitative research. Qualitative Health Research 11 (4): 117–132.

Winter, G. (2000). A comparative discussion of the notion of "validity" in qualitative and quantitative research. The Qualitative Report 4 (3): 1–14.

Yin, R.K. (1994). Discovering the future of the case study method in evaluation research. Evaluation Practice 15 (3): 283–290.

IV

The Art of Phenomenological Writing, Reporting, and Publishing

6

Qualitative Phenomenological Writing

The final stage of a phenomenological research endeavor is crafting and creating the "write-up." The completed research should advance knowledge and be of interest to the scientific community. Thus, the results are written-up and published (Morse and Field 1995). The researcher, who at this point is equipped with some explicated meanings, sits down to write and becomes aware of some of the challenges ahead: achieving a degree of scientific credibility, expressing the phenomenon evocatively, and integrating phenomenological concepts within the writing (Finlay 2014). Human science research is a form of writing (van Manen 1990). Writing is not just the last step of the research process, or about writing up study results. It is also a way of "knowing" – a method of discovery and analysis (Denzin and Lincoln 1994). Creating a phenomenological text is the object of the research process. It is a reflective part of the interpretive phenomenological method (van Manen 1990, 2014). To do research in a phenomenological sense is already, immediately, and always to bring to speech or to writing (van Manen 1990). What is the phenomenon of writing? What does it mean to write phenomenologically? Van Manen (2014) argues:

> I am vaguely aware that the experience of writing (or trying to write) something happens to me. I seem to be seeking a certain space. A writerly space. In this space, I am no longer quite myself. Just as in reading a compelling story, the self of the reader seems to have slipped away, so in the act of writing the "self" has become partially erased. It is like falling into a twilight zone, where there are no longer recognizable the same, where words are displaced, where you can lose your orientation, where anything can happen. Is this what makes writing difficult; the sense of erasure of the self? Should I actively and reflectively seek to write? Or should I seek to surrender myself to that special reflective mood? I type, "phenomenological reflecting is already like writing in the sense that we withdraw from the world." (p. 358)

Writing is not just putting into language the spoken words. It is being inside the thoughts in which you dwell in an inner space, inside the self – or what van Manen (2014) calls "in the textorium," the virtual space that the words open up. In other words,

Fundamentals of Qualitative Phenomenological Nursing Research, First Edition. Brigitte S. Cypress.
© 2022 John Wiley & Sons Ltd. Published 2022 by John Wiley & Sons Ltd.

we are using a spatial/temporal phenomenology (van Manen 2014). It is a temporal experience in the world evoked by the words of the text that phenomenologists experience. To write is a solitary experience, a self-forgetful submersion in textual reality that one traverses through language until insights occur. The world of text has obscurity, shadow and darkness that make it impossible to write – yet, one must write; one has become one who writes (van Manen 2014, p. 359). The words draw the writer in once writing begins, and one finds one's starting point in wonder. For a phenomenological text to lead the way to human understanding, it must lead the reader to wonder. One also adopts a relation to language that is reflective. It is the minded act of writing that orients itself to a notion that is a feature of lived experience. Phenomenological research requires a commitment to write. The writer produces more than text: they also produce themselves (van Manen 2014). Van Manen articulates that "the writer is the product of his or her own product. Writing is a kind of self-making or forming. To write is to measure the depth of things, as well as to come to a sense of one's own depth" (p. 365).

Phenomenological inquiry cannot be separated from the practice of writing. Phenomenological reflection is writing. The research *is* the writing (van Manen 2014). It is in the act of reading and writing that insights emerge. Writing involves textual material that possesses hermeneutic and interpretive significance, and through which the fundamental nature of the research questions is perceived. In the phenomenological sense, knowledge is produced from the research in the form of texts. These texts explore, describe, and evoke understanding phenomena of the lifeworld. Writing thus creates a space that belongs to the unpresentable. It is bringing into presence a phenomenon that cannot be represented in plain words. Language substitutes itself for the phenomenon that it tries to describe – but qualitative method as writing is not easy. It is often difficult, and it requires interpretive skills and creative talents from the researcher (van Manen 2014).

Writing that truly addresses the meaning of something is an entitled endeavor that can be claimed by a talented author and scholar. So, if the goal of writing is to touch something meaningful, then this is no privileged pursuit. Van Manen (2014) states: "Writing is not something with which we make peace. Rather, one learns to obey its demand with the hope of an uncertain promise: to satisfy the desire really to 'write' something, to see what we try to write in its nakedness" (p. 373). Reluctance to write is common in student writers. In the beginning, they may need encouragement. The student writer practices writing in the hope of making something clear. Once a real desire to write is ignited, no encouragement is needed. To write is to be driven by desire, and thus one has become a real writer propelled to cross the space of the texts, and the true nature of writing can reveal itself (van Manen 2014).

6.1 Ethical Considerations in Writing

Before delving into the approaches to and techniques of qualitative phenomenological writing, relevant ethical considerations must first be discussed. A qualitative researcher must adhere to and comply with appropriate reporting strategies and ethical publishing practices. These include the use of appropriate language for the target audience, writing

Table 6.1 Ethical writing questions for qualitative researchers.

- Have I obtained permission for use of unpublished procedures or data that other researchers might consider their proprietary?
- Have I properly cited other published work presented in portions of the manuscript?
- Am I prepared to answer questions about institutional review of my study or studies?
- Am I prepared to answer editorial questions about the informed consent and debriefing procedures used in the study?
- Have all authors reviewed the manuscript and agreed on the responsibility for its content? (if with co-authors)
- Have I adequately protected the confidentiality of research participants, clients-patients, third parties, or others who were the source of information presented in the manuscript?
- Have all authors agreed to the order of authorship? (if with co-authors)
- Have I obtained permission for use of copyrighted material included?

Source: Creswell, J. W. & Poth, C. N. (2017). *Qualitative Inquiry & Research Design: Choosing Among Five Approaches*, 4th ed., Sage Publications.

reports that are honest and trustworthy, seeking permissions as needed, and disclosing funders or any conflicts of interest. Creswell (2016) presents a checklist adapted from the American Psychological Association of questions that need to be asked by all qualitative researchers, as given in Table 6.1.

6.2 Approaches in Qualitative Writing

6.2.1 Getting Started

The first step in writing is to clearly identify what you have to say and to whom you wish to say it. You must be ready before beginning to write. The analysis or theoretical work must be finished (Morse and Field 1995). You must be clear about the purpose of the writing, and identify the audience you intend the writing for (Morse and Field 1995; Patton 2015). It can be an article for a journal, a monograph, a dissertation, or another form of writing. Creswell and Poth (2018) present four approaches in qualitative writing as a whole: reflexivity and representation, audience, encoding, and quotes.

6.2.2 Reflexivity and Representation

Analysis and reporting are where reflexivity comes to the fore (Patton 2015). The writing of qualitative text cannot be separated from the author, how it is received by readers, and how it impacts the participants and sites under study. Qualitative researchers need to "position" themselves in their writing, engaging in self-understanding about the biases, values, and experiences that they bring to a naturalistic inquiry. How we write is a reflection of our own interpretations based on the cultural, social, gender, class, and personal politics that we bring to research (Creswell and Poth 2018). Reflexivity is about the researcher recognizing their experiences with the phenomenon being explored and discussing how they shape their findings, conclusions, and interpretation.

Qualitative writers are the sole instruments of their studies that shape the writing that emerges, and are open to co-constructions, representation of interactive processes, and interpretations between researchers and the participants. They are not separate from the participants and the readers (Creswell and Poth 2018). Patton (2015) emphasizes that the following self-reflexivity questions should be asked: What do I know? How do I know what I know? What has shaped my perspective? How have my perceptions and background affected the data I have collected and my analysis of those data? How do I perceive those I have studied? With what voice do I share my perspective? What do I do with what I found? (p. 604). Aside from reflexivity and representation, the impact of the writing to the participants should also be considered (Creswell and Poth 2018).

Creswell and Poth (2018) articulate that from the perspective of the study participants, these questions should be regarded: How will they see the write-up? Will they be marginalized because of it? Will they be offended? Will they hide their true feelings and perspectives? Have the participants reviewed the material and interpreted, challenged, and dissented from the interpretation? Similarly, Patton (2015) advocates for the questions: How do those studied know what they know? What had shaped their worldview? How do they perceive me, the inquirer? Why? How do I know?

Impact on the readers also needs to be considered. Thus, the following questions have to be taken into account: Should the researcher be afraid that certain people will see the final report? Can the researcher give any kind of definitive account when it is the reader who makes the ultimate interpretation of the events? (Creswell and Poth 2018). Patton (2015) adds the following: How do those who receive my findings make sense of what I give them? What perspectives do they bring to the findings I offer? How do they perceive me? How do I perceive them? How do these perceptions affect what I report and how I report it? (p. 605).

6.2.3 Audience

All writers write for an audience (Creswell and Poth 2018). Identifying the target audience helps inform choices during the writing process. This means that a report is structured according to the readers the researcher wants to engage in the writing. Creswell and Poth (2018) state that the following questions should be taken into account: For what audience is this study being written? What informs these choices? What am I hoping to achieve with this report to my audience? What writing structures should my audience expect? Are there other audiences who could benefit from my learning and knowledge? How might I structure my writing to fit the other audiences' needs?

6.2.4 Encoding

Language is important in shaping a qualitative report. The words qualitative researchers use encode their texts (Creswell and Poth 2018). Encoding an entire qualitative narrative includes an overall structure that does not follow a quantitative format (e.g., making headings about themes in the study findings, calling "methods" the "procedures"). The writing style has to be personal, familiar, highly readable, friendly, persuasive, and in first-person active voice. It should also be "real" and "alive," transporting the reader directly into the world of the study (Creswell and Poth 2018).

6.2.5 Quotes

The voice of the participants in the study should come alive through the use of quotes that are as illustrative as possible, contextualized, interpreted, and incorporated within the text of the manuscript (Creswell and Poth 2018). Quotes supplement the text, and provide human insight and dimension to the analysis (Morse and Field 1995). They should be easy to read, stand out from the narrator's text, and be indented to signify different perspectives. For example, in the phenomenological study of Cypress (2010), the patients conveyed "transformation" as a theme by saying:

> Being critically ill in the ICU was scary because you don't know where your life is going to go or if you're going to live, or you're going to die. It was scary just not knowing what is going to go on. I was surprised; all this stuff happened to me like in one day. I was happy one hour, and then the next hour, I'm in the hospital. Being in a position like this, everything is spontaneous you don't know what's going to happen. (p. 99)

6.3 Phenomenological Writing

A human science phenomenological study needs rich experiential material to be successful. Whatever method of writing up is used, the key is to try to capture the complexity and ambiguity of the lived world being described (Finlay 2014). How can we develop rich descriptions faithful to the phenomenon that evoke the ambiguously lived embodied world? How can we enact both scientific and communicative concerns? (Finlay 2014). Concrete, active, first-person descriptions of lived experience are often the starting point for phenomenological reflection and exploration in published human science studies (Adams and van Manen 2018). The aim of first-person phenomenological approaches is to provide rich, compelling, and thought-provoking descriptions of lived experience (Finlay 2012). The voices of the participants must be heard from the texts (Beck 2021).

6.3.1 Strategies

Those who write phenomenology should provide considerable attention to the different strategies available: anecdotal or "story," use of metaphor, reflexivity using existential methods, incorporating visuals, and use of figures, diagrams, models, and tables.

6.3.1.1 Anecdotal or "Story"

One strategy in phenomenological writing is to use anecdotal narrative or "story." Anecdotes are a special kind of story that make comprehensible some notion that easily eludes us (van Manen 1990). The story or narrative form is one of the most popular methods for presenting aspects of human science research. Adams and van Manen (2018) describe this as "anecdote/reflection" – a way of writing phenomenologically. The anecdote/reflection pair consists of a carefully crafted lived experience description followed closely by a reflection on an aspect or aspects of the phenomenon given in the anecdote.

Anecdotes may get negative reactions as it is entirely fallacious to generalize from a case on the basis of mere anecdotal evidence. However, empirical generalization is not the aim of phenomenological research. The object is not to develop theoretical abstractions but to try and penetrate the layers of meaning and lay bare lived experience (van Manen 1990). The significance of anecdotal narrative in phenomenological research and writing is its power to compel. It leads us to reflect, involves us personally, transforms us, and shows a measure of our interpretive sense (van Manen 1990). I will illustrate the use of anecdotal narrative or storytelling in a qualitative study with the following example.

Bourbonnais and Michaud (2018) illustrated the potential of storytelling as a knowledge translation strategy in healthcare during a qualitative study in a nursing home. Their story began with a narration by a fictional older person, who screamed:

> *Sometimes, I feel bored and even like I am dead already. I am always so glad when you come talk to me! I open my arms invitingly. I am always happy when my daughter visits, too. I don't always remember her name or even remember she is my daughter, but I am always pleased to see her. When she says I am screaming, I'm surprised. I am not always aware of doing it. It must be very puzzling to her but, honestly, I don't know why I do it. My screams seem to be disturbing because people avoid me. Some even become angry when I scream, but I really don't mean to bother anyone. (p. 5)*

To empower the nurses' aides who were already very engaged in understanding the meanings of the patient, they read this story to their co-workers during a training workshop for clinicians and at a conference. They realized that this knowledge translation strategy raised listeners'/readers' awareness of older people's experience. It also triggered dialogue and helped them understand the usefulness of the intervention. By showing the usefulness of qualitative studies' results, storytelling truly reduces the gap between research and practice (Bourbonnais and Michaud 2018).

6.3.1.2 Use of Metaphor

Metaphor is the backbone of social science writing (Denzin and Lincoln 1994). Metaphors are generally considered figures of speech, but they are more important than that. They give important clues about how an individual sees/perceives life, their environment, events, and objects. They allow the individual to see a certain fact as another fact by directing their mind from one perception form to another. This means that metaphors not only influence thought processes, language, and science, but also have a formative effect on the way individuals express themselves (Senyuva and Kaya 2013). The use of metaphor can be a powerful way of connecting to readers of qualitative research (Patton 2015). It is chiefly a tool for revealing special properties of an object or event. Its use should serve the data and not vice versa. In other words, do not manipulate the data to fit the metaphor. Patton (2015) states: "because metaphors carry implicit connotation, it is important to make sure that the data fit the most prominent of those connotations so that what is communicated is what the analysts wants to communicate" (p. 607). I will illustrate the use of metaphor in the following example.

A study by Senyuva and Kaya (2013) regarding nursing students' perceptions of the Internet through metaphors found that the predominant categories were: the Internet as a source of information, as a harmful tool, as both useful and harmful, and as a comprehensive tool. When these conceptual categories were examined, it was seen that the category "the Internet as a harmful tool" consisted of 44 metaphors produced by 109 students. The most common metaphors for Internet use in this category were drug, cigarette, alcohol, virus, spider's web, love, and addiction. Senyuva and Kaya (2013) presented their participants' statements as follows:

> *Internet is like alcohol that it causes addiction over time . . . Internet is like a spider's web. When you get caught, it is difficult to escape, and it is a system where you waste time for nothing . . . Internet is like a drug. It gives you pleasure and joy when you first start it. With time, it becomes an indispensable part of your life. You think you use it because you want it. (p. 97)*

6.3.1.3 Reflexivity Using Existential Methods

The phenomenological researcher can engage their writing in a dialogue with that of others (like philosophers) and weave in descriptions of time, space, the lived body, and their lived relation with others (based on Merleau-Ponty's existentials). This is a creative way of expressing the meaning of a phenomenon that is considered reflective phenomenological research-writing. According to van Manen (1990, 2014), the phenomenon at hand can be explored by placing it in the context of the four existentials. These existentials illustrate a fusion of the objectivist hermeneutic circle (part-whole) and the alethic hermeneutic circle (pre-understanding) as they acknowledge the experience of a phenomenon in a whole experience and the researcher's role in the research process. A full exemplar of the use of Merleau-Ponty's four existentials is presented in Chapter 2.

6.3.1.4 Incorporating Visuals

The best way to present qualitative data visualization is not to talk about visuals but to provide actual illustrations (Patton 2015). Usually, the center of a qualitative data analysis is words from narratives, documents, and stories – but pictures, visuals, and graphics are worth a thousand words (Patton 2015). Florence Nightingale, for example, gathered data during the Crimean War and converted them into color-coded visual displays that proved highly influential in changing sanitation practices and paved the way for attention to preventing infections (Patton 2015, p. 608).

6.3.1.5 Use of Figures, Diagrams, Models, and Tables

The representation of qualitative data is enhanced by the use of figures, diagrams, models, and tables. These visuals provide overviews and schemes of the study (Morse and Field 1995). They also help summarize key findings and bring the results to life (Beck 2021). For readers of a phenomenological study, for example, figures, diagrams, and tables help to break up page after page of text. Another advantage is that they make it easier to meet the page limitations of a journal to which the researcher plans to submit their manuscript (Beck 2021).

Two examples are presented here from my published phenomenological studies in the intensive care unit (**ICU**) and emergency department (**ED**). Figure 6.1 is about the

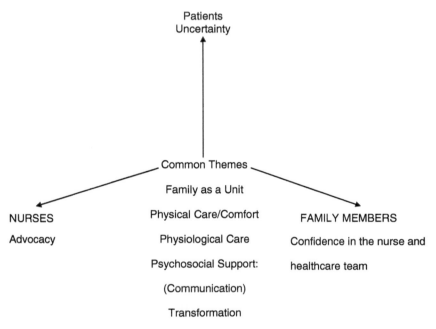

Figure 6.1 Patient–family–nurse lived ICU experiences themes and descriptors. Source: Based on Cypress, B. S. (2013). Using the synergy model of patient care in understanding the lived emergency department experiences of patients, family members and their nurses during critical illness. *Dimensions of Critical Care Nursing*, 32(6): 310–321.

lived experiences of nurses, patients, and family members during critical illness in the ICU. It illustrates five integrating common themes and three specific themes illuminated in the study. These themes constitute the perceived experiences of patients and family members cared for by nurses during critical illness in the ICU. Each has specific descriptors. Figure 6.2 presents the findings of my phenomenological research into the lived experiences of nurses, patients, and family members during critical illness in the ED. Five essential themes and corresponding descriptors emerged from the thematic analysis of the participants' narratives, constituting the perceived experiences of nurses, patients, and family members in the ED setting.

6.3.2 Practicing How to Write Phenomenologically

Van Manen (2014) presents suggestions on how one may practice writing phenomenologically through heuristic, experiential, thematic, vocative, and insight-cultivating writing. Heuristic draft writing involves invoking wonder in the reader through the writing of a single or a few small paragraphs. This is challenging and difficult to do. Experiential draft writing involves inserting lived experiences into the text. This can be done using anecdotes, examples, fragments, and stories that embody the phenomenon at hand. Thematic writing involves examining experiential aspects of the phenomenon

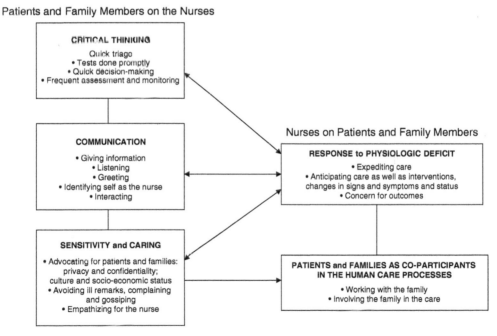

Patients and Family Members on the Nurses

CRITICAL THINKING

Quick triage
• Tests done promptly
• Quick decision-making
• Frequent assessment and monitoring

COMMUNICATION

• Giving information
• Listening
• Greeting
• Identifying self as the nurse
• Interacting

Nurses on Patients and Family Members

RESPONSE to PHYSIOLOGIC DEFICIT

• Expediting care
• Anticipating care as well as interventions, changes in signs and symptoms and status
• Concern for outcomes

SENSITIVITY and CARING

• Advocating for patients and families: privacy and confidentiality; culture and socio-economic status
• Avoiding ill remarks, complaining and gossiping
• Empathizing for the nurse

PATIENTS and FAMILIES AS CO-PARTICIPANTS IN THE HUMAN CARE PROCESSES

• Working with the family
• Involving the family in the care

Figure 6.2 Patient–family–nurse lived ED experiences themes and descriptors. Source: Based on Cypress, B. S. (2013). Using the synergy model of patient care in understanding the lived emergency department experiences of patients, family members and their nurses during critical illness. *Dimensions of Critical Care Nursing*, 32(6): 310–321.

under study. It might begin with an essence description, and then present varying examples of how the essence is manifested. Thematic draft writing goes hand in hand with experiential writing. Themes are succinct phrasings that are discerned during analysis of the concrete or experiential material. Vocative draft writing involves tactful attentiveness to the vocative nature of language – a part of the phenomenological writing process. Vocative writing aims for texts to speak to our whole embodied being through eloquent integration of anecdotes, examples, and selective material from literature, art, and mythology. Insight-cultivating draft writing is enabled by reflections on sources that draw on other scholarly phenomenological texts or which are gleaned metaphorically from relevant literature.

6.4 Writing and Rewriting

In teaching phenomenological research to graduate students and novices of this area of inquiry, I emphasize (from van Manen's 1990 words) that phenomenology as a method of inquiry is "more a cultivated thoughtfulness than a technique." Van Manen (1990) asserts that in order to do justice to the fullness and ambiguity of the experience of the lifeworld, writing may turn into a complex process of rewriting. In other words, it is an ongoing practice of writing and rewriting (Adams and van Manen 2018). Van Manen (1990) states:

> the process of writing and rewriting (including revising and editing) is more reminiscent of the artistic activity of creating an art object that has to be approached again and again, now here and then there, going back and forth between the parts and the whole in order to arrive at a finely crafted piece that often reflects the personal "signature" of the author. (p. 132)

It is only in the process of rewriting that phenomenological insights are attained (Adams and van Manen 2018). Novices and students of phenomenological inquiry should be supported, guided, mentored, and encouraged in honing their skills in writing, rewriting, and reflecting. Adams and van Manen (2018) articulate that this can be done by giving writing exercises with a set of criteria when teaching phenomenological research and assigning them in writing groups. Drafts of individual papers should be read and discussed by the whole seminar group. Everyone learns in this process, and eventually the class gains experience in writing lived experience descriptions, interviewing one another, crafting anecdotes, analyzing experiential materials thematically and existentially, writing reflectively and vocatively, and appraising phenomenological texts (Adams and van Manen 2018).

6.5 Conclusion

This chapter discussed the importance of writing as a step in phenomenological research. Ethical considerations, approaches in qualitative writing, the different structures and modes of presenting narrative texts and other visuals, and reflexivity and rewriting were described. The significance of mentoring students to write, rewrite, and reflect as they go through these steps was also examined.

References

Adams, C. and van Manen, M.A. (2018). Teaching phenomenological research and writing. Qualitative Health Research 27 (6): 780–791.

Beck, C. (2021). Introduction to Phenomenology: Focus on Methodology. Sage Publications.

Bourbonnais, A. and Michaud, C. (2018). Once upon a time: storytelling as a knowledge translation strategy for qualitative researchers. Nursing Inquiry 25: e12249.

Creswell, J.W. (2016). 30 Essential Skills for Qualitative Researcher. Sage Publications.

Creswell, J.W. and Poth, C.N. (2018). Qualitative Inquiry and Research Design: Choosing among Five Approaches. Sage Publications.

Cypress, B. (2010). The intensive care unit: experiences of patients, families, and their nurses. Dimensions of Critical Care Nursing 29 (2): 94–101.

Denzin, N. and Lincoln, Y.S. (1994). Handbook of Qualitative Research. Sage Publications.

Finlay, L. (2012). "Writing the pain": engaging firs-person phenomenological accounts. Indo-Pacific Journal of Phenomenology 12 (Special edition): 1–9.

Finlay L. (2014). Writing up and evaluating phenomenological findings. Available from http://lindafinlay.co.uk/wp-content/uploads/2014/05/Writing-up-and-evaluating-phenomenological-findings.pdf (accessed May 10, 2021).

Morse, J. and Field, P.A. (1995). Qualitative Research Methods for Health Professionals. Sage Publications.

Patton, M.Q. (2015). Qualitative Research and Valuation Methods, 4e. Sage Publications.

Senyuva, E. and Kaya, H. (2013). Metaphors for the Internet used by nursing students in Turkey: a qualitative research. Eurasian Journal of Educational Research 50: 87–106.

van Manen, M. (1990). Researching Lived Experience: Human Science for an Action Sensitive Pedagogy. State University Press.

van Manen, M. (2014). Phenomenology of Practice: Meaning-Giving Methods in Phenomenological Research and Writing. Left Coast Press.

7 Publishing Qualitative Phenomenological Research Findings

Kathleen Ahern Gould

Researchers are scientists, and science requires communication and writing skills to move it forward. Professional publication can be a daunting task even for the most experienced investigator. Dissemination of findings of qualitative research has never been more important. As members of a practice profession providing evidence-based care, all healthcare disciplines need knowledge that is scientific, experiential, and practical. Publishing in a scholarly journal is a very efficient way to share this knowledge. Publication is a fundamental vehicle that closes the gap between conducting a study and presenting results that move practice forward and consequently improve patient outcomes (Gennaro 2018).

When embarking on a research project, there are many objectives to consider. As a timeline is established, one early goal should involve dissemination of the completed work. Scholarly work can be disseminated locally, nationally, and globally. Each way of communicating research findings may serve a specific or diverse audience, yet it also informs other methods. As the study plan evolves, there are many details that may direct steps toward publication. Thus, this process should be taken into consideration from early on.

7.1 Publication of Qualitative Research

Qualitative research crosses many disciplines and offers a wide variety of approaches. It is classified very differently from quantitative research. Naturalistic investigations may be categorized more by disciplinary traditions or inquiry frameworks, which often serve for the theoretical underpinning for the study (Polit and Beck 2021). Often, qualitative research is the best way to build knowledge about the experience of individuals or to explore a phenomenon of interest. One of the long-standing tenets of qualitative descriptive study is that a wide net should be cast to gather a breadth of data from multiple sources in order to describe experiences (Sandelowski 1995). This type of research is widely applied in the social sciences, and has evolved into an important design for all disciplines in healthcare. Key stakeholders in nursing broadly support qualitative research to enrich the acquisition of new knowledge. As research methodologies continue to mature, qualitative research has added a new dimension to the

Fundamentals of Qualitative Phenomenological Nursing Research, First Edition. Brigitte S. Cypress.
© 2022 John Wiley & Sons Ltd. Published 2022 by John Wiley & Sons Ltd.

patient perspective and to the scope of population health. Professional publication allows a venue to disseminate this unique form of knowledge.

Conducting qualitative research is a complex, tedious, and difficult endeavor for researchers at every stage of their professional development, and especially for students and novice researchers (Cypress 2018). Qualitative data is also complex, multidimensional, and derived from natural settings with specific designs that help communicate findings (Cypress 2020). This process requires support and education. Mentorship at each stage is essential, yet it does not always include a writing coach or editor. Doctoral students working with a nurse scientist or professor serving as a committee chair may have an advantage, as both have expertise in professional publication. Often, there are many personal and professional incentives that provide structure and opportunity for dissemination of work through posters, podium presentations, and abstract publication. With the right mentor and resources, these formats can translate into key steps within the publication. Cypress provides an in-depth discussion about mentorship in qualitative research in Chapter 9 of this current work. As a skilled phenomenologist, she combines her knowledge and experience to guide the novice and advanced qualitative researcher alike. Her detailed descriptions and unique understanding of phenomenology will be helpful to those writing a qualitative research proposal, report, or manuscript (Cypress 2017, 2018, 2020). This chapter provides publishing resources and advice for both new and experienced qualitative researchers that will help them move toward professional publication of their scholarly work.

7.1.1 Why Publish?

Oermann and Hays (2016) describe five main reasons to write for publication: (i) to share ideas and expertise with other nurses; (ii) to disseminate evidence and the findings of nursing research studies; (iii) for promotion, tenure, and other personnel decisions; (iv) for development of one's knowledge and skills; and, finally, (v) for one's personal satisfaction. Many researchers have more than one reason to publish. Some may have all five, and some other additional individual motivations besides. Yet, researchers and writers share the same fears and limitations. Writing may be a new form of communication or something that existed in a remote past. It is a skill that must be nurtured and practiced, but certainly it is one that can be enhanced at any stage of life. Becoming a published author and a successful writer does require that one possess an understanding of publication ethics and attends to the obligations of authorship and the fundamentals of the publishing process. Additionally, it requires the ability to apply the basic rules of writing, such as composition, grammar, syntax, and style. All of these can be learned, relearned, and improved upon.

Writing is hard work, often solitary, and exhausting. Professional publication can be intimidating. Many professionals who publish engage or employ writing coaches, join writing groups, or add steps to the research process that enhance the chances of their manuscript receiving a final acceptance in a scholarly journal. Much of this is very accessible, and many authors and editors share their knowledge freely. Chin (2014) reminds us that the truth is that there are no real secrets. All those articles and books about the writing process really do reveal just about all there is to know! The problem is not a lack of knowledge about the writing process. There are some barriers, but most can be easily tackled with commitment and hard work. For many authors, the real challenges are the nuances of electronic resources, submission procedures, and timely publication. Often, the problems are inspiration, motivation, and dedication (Chin 2014).

The publishing journey is an extended process. It requires a strategic plan and is informed by logistics that address each step. Finding a journal, textbook, or format for new writing requires some working knowledge of the state of scientific publishing and some idea about the dissemination of research. Information on these topics is widely available in published texts, articles, and digital formats.

7.2 First Steps: Authorship

If the goal is to pursue publication, it may take some time to finalize authorship agreements. If more than one author will be involved in publication, it is best to make some agreements early – perhaps even before communication with potential publishers begins. A longstanding recommendation from the Committee on Publication Ethics (COPE 2018, 2021) advises discussing authorship at the beginning of a research project. This discussion should capture the views of all team members. Authorship should be presented as a standalone topic, preferably at a face-to-face meeting. Often, the group will have some idea of the publications or presentations that might disseminate its study. This might include conference abstracts, an abstract or full paper, some supplementary papers, podium presentations, a podcast, or social media formats. A discussion about authorship can direct many of these assignments and clarify who is likely to be involved in each opportunity. As the project evolves, the researchers may continue to discuss ideas about authorship, especially if new people get involved and additional formats become available. A written record of your decisions will be helpful and may serve as a template for adjustments and changes that will aid with final decisions later (Albert and Wagner 2003).

7.2.1 Authorship Agreements

Normally, the individual who is the primary investigator or who has served as the leader in research design, data generation and analysis, and in writing the article itself will be the first author. Research teams usually determine authorship based on levels of contribution. Publications resulting from student projects should have the student as first author. Professors and supervising personnel may be first authors only if they meet the criteria of authorship and are acknowledged as such by the leading writer (COPE 2018, 2021; ICMJE 2021). Acknowledgments can be added at the end of the publication to recognize others who have contributed to the work but are not listed as authors.

Authorship controversies are not uncommon, but they can be painful and potentially harmful to personal and professional relationships. Many authorship difficulties are not ethically induced, but simply arise because of misplaced expectations and poor communication. Authors working with friends or colleagues often make assumptions based on their relationship. It is important to remember that co-authorship is a different relationship. It is an ethical and a professional contract. When friends, colleagues, and power relationships are involved, an early, candid discussion about authorship is in everyone's best interest. This is not a problem with single authors. Work involving more than one author requires clarification of roles before or as the search for a journal begins. Collaboration with colleagues, peers, and even friends is a true strength during the publication process. However, there are times when even the most successful friendships and relationships need clarification and definition. Authorship is one of these times.

Journals' definitions as to what constitutes authorship may vary, although biomedical journals are guided by ethical guidelines provided by the International Council of Medical Journal Editors (ICMJE 2021) and COPE (2018, 2021). These groups are committed to educating and supporting authors, editors, publishers, and those involved in publication ethics. Free resources may be obtained directly through their websites, and are often linked to in journal guidelines. It is helpful to review these resources before and during authorship discussions as they are specific to the complexities often woven into scientific research and collaboration.

The concept of authorship should be straightforward. Scientific research commonly involves others. Authorship may be one way to recognize people's contributions and acknowledge them for their work within a study or final product. Often, published works list the contributions of each author and verify the continued application of work through to the final revision process. Authorship confounds everyone involved in writing. Publication relationships are challenging, as they often involve the inherent power dynamics of work relationships (Hein and Chin 2017). To begin a discussion, first consider who launched the idea, who is inviting other authors, and who was the first to put pen to paper or fingers to keyboard. These first steps may be the basis for more formal discussion about qualifications for authorship and the order of co-authors.

7.2.2 Student Authors

Students who are reporting the results of their independent research or individual projects should be first author of their hard work. Students will often ask if it is appropriate, required, or necessary to include faculty as co-authors. This decision is up to the student. Faculty or colleagues who read, edit, or approve a paper may not meet the criteria defined by the ICMJE or COPE for authorship. The student may choose to invite any person who has made a substantial contribution to the manuscript. Others who have guided the work may be formally acknowledged at the end of the paper. Student authors have much to consider when transforming schoolwork, including state-of-the-science papers, quality improvement work, and evidence-based projects, dissertations, or capstone projects. All of these may be transformed into a scholarly work that is publishable.

7.3 Finding the Right Journal

There are many formats in which to disseminate one's work. Finding the right journal may feel like more of a "Goldilocks" process than a scholarly one. The right journal might be a "good fit" for the topic, the audience, the profession, or the author themselves. The search may be guided by a host of factors, some personal, others professional. Finding the right fit takes some time and investigation. It may also involve communication with administrative or academic colleagues, or with a publishing professional, editor, editorial board member, or experienced published author.

Ideally, the work of finding the right journal should begin as the project is developed, not when the reporting and writing commences. This is because each journal has specific guidelines, formats, and requirements that must be adhered to prior to publication. Preparing a research project with this specific information in hand helps in including details of rigor and methods within the study design, execution, and reporting of data. Individual publishers provide specific guidelines for each type of research study and manuscript preparation. These are extremely helpful for publication, but also serve as a checklist for rigorous methodological management of the study. Compliance with a journal format, including reference style, manuscript length, and use of stylistic points and tone, indicates that the author has directed the work to the specific journal. The writer should also read and incorporate the information for authors (IFA), which is specific to each journal. This may contribute to the advancement of the manuscript toward possible acceptance. Failure to adhere to these guidelines could mean early rejection; alternatively, the manuscript will need reformatting to meet the requirements outlined in the IFA documents if it is to advance further in the publication process. Editors may move a manuscript through technical checks, and possibly to peer review. Editorial consideration could be more favorable to authors who have attended to the requirements of the journal.

7.3.1 Personal Goals, Options, and Professional Requirements

The right journal will be one that meets the authors' specific requirements. Some authors may freely choose the journal they wish to submit to – based on their professional knowledge and personal associations. Others will be directed by criteria defined by their employers. Professional prestige, organizational sponsorship, scope, or impact may be the drivers of this decision, as journal metrics vary and remain a source of controversy. In the quest for the right journal, it is important to ask about acceptance rates and publication timelines.

7.3.2 Choosing or Selecting a Journal

Journal selection is similar to selecting a college. The search process is similar, and the outcomes are almost identical. In the end, the goal is a "good fit." However, as with the college search process, selection does not ensure acceptance! Unlike when applying to college, you may not submit your work to many journals and hope for an acceptance. Each manuscript must be submitted to only one journal at a time. Subsequent submission may be commenced only after rejection or withdrawal from the selected journal. To encourage and ensure this behavior, many publishers require copyright agreements to be completed at the time of submission. Some submission sites ask authors to confirm that the manuscript has not been submitted elsewhere. This is an important ethical consideration in professional publishing. For this reason, a targeted approach to manuscript submission is important to an efficient and timely publication.

The list of biomedical journals is extensive. More and more nursing journals are appearing, and many specialty journals encourage work from complementary disciplines and multidisciplinary research. There are thus a great number of choices and options. Qualitative research is accepted in many journals. It should not be limited to qualitative research journals, as the topic or phenomenon of interest may inform clinical, educational, leadership, or specialty journals. Indeed, qualitative design is needed in every forum, as it may serve as a basis for future research, provide cross-discipline definitions, and help identify new concepts, clinical issues, and ways of understanding individual patients and populations. It is important to remind all potential authors and qualitative researcher teams to expand their journal search beyond qualitative, research-only, or topic-specific journals.

Once you have a journal in mind, contact the editor or an editorial board member to ask questions about it. Take the opportunity to introduce yourself and your study purpose. Often, this is done in the form of a query letter, sent by email directly to the editor or to the editorial office. It is also helpful to work with a librarian and to network with published authors, editors, academics, and colleagues. They may identify resources that will help expand your search. To expedite this process, the International Academy of Nursing Editors (INANE) has curated and vetted a list of over 200 nursing journals, with a goal of helping nurse authors find suitable and reputable journals in which to publish their work. Recently, the list was converted into a visual digital format using air table technology (INANE n.d.).

7.3.3 Solicited Authorship

It is quite common for journals and editors to invite expert clinicians and researchers to submit work. Often, this occurs when the work is presented in a local forum, national or international conference, or poster presentation, or when it is mentioned in conference proceedings during a podium presentation. It is not unusual for an editor or someone connected to a professional publication to approach the presenter to discuss a possible publication. This type of invitation is exciting and encouraging for researchers at all levels. It often leads to a timely publication if all steps of the publication process, including peer reviews, are completed successfully. However, authors must check the journal and ensure that it is a valid scholarly publication and a "good fit" for their work.

7.3.4 Predatory Journals and Publishers

A discussion about solicitation must include a discussion about predatory publishing. A common form of solicitation is that from predatory journals and publishers. It is important to know that predatory publishers may contact people with offers for speedy publication and open access (OA) for a fee. Predatory (as the word implies) publishers prey on unsuspecting authors, luring them with offers of quick turnaround times for fees often ranging into thousands of dollars. Most reputable scholarly journals do not offer payment for articles in this manner, but may contract with authors for gold or green OA. This issue is discussed later in this chapter. However, reimbursement for chapter and book publication is common. Some due diligence is required for any solicited work.

INANE supports research and updates on this topic, as the open-access model has encouraged opportunistic and predatory behaviors to flourish, and the quality of articles in predatory journals remains questionable (Oermann et al. 2018a).

As one investigates the validity of a journal or publisher, it is important to know that many predatory operations are well funded and appear to be valid. Often, their names will be quite similar to those of well-recognized publications, with letterheads, banners, and logos that may also appear familiar and valid. However, upon further investigation, it will often be difficult to find the publisher's address, leadership board, or other reputable identifiers. A reputable journal will be easily assessable, will identify its editor and editorial board members, and will respond freely to questions and concerns from the potential author. Many published authors receive unsolicited invitations from all types of journals, but beware of those that invite you to send checks, money orders, or electronic payments with your submission, without a clear contract agreement for gold or green OA. It is prudent to investigate all invitations, but especially those that request payment in the early stages. Predators in this space prey on those eager to publish, and often those under professional scrutiny to produce scholarly work. Tenure committees and professional organizations do not recognize such work.

7.3.5 Non-traditional Publishing Formats

Perhaps a traditional journal does not meet the immediate needs of your work. A timelier option might be a poster, podcast, or blog. These formats can be selected and later referenced, if copyright applies, for a more traditional journal article. The traditional publication model is changing for all disciplines. Digital formats command center stage as print and hard-copy journals are in transition, although they are still considered the "gold standard" for many professionals. During the search for the right journal or format, be aware that publishing houses change names and acquire existing journals, adding some confusion to the hunt for a perfect fit. Traditional science journals will not disappear, but the options for publication have certainly changed. We have barely scratched the surface of what digital technology, social media, and all forms of visual media will mean for scholarly communications. Many publishers have merged traditional and novel formats and may offer authors several options to extend dissemination of their work.

Publishing in preprint format is another option. Preprints are part of a research project or completed research that has not yet been peer-reviewed or published in a peer review journal. Often, they are working drafts or pre-released papers, which may be valuable but lack the scientific rigor that is assigned through the peer review process – the hallmark of scientific publication.

7.3.6 Journal Quality and Metrics

The norm is for authors to publish in a peer-reviewed journal. Peer-reviewed journals are also called refereed journals, and adhere to the standards of scientific peer review. Both quality and metrics may play a role in journal selection. However, metrics are not always an indicator of journal or article quality. Journal-level metrics are indicators of how widely a journal is used. Article-level metrics indicate readership through digital tracking and communications. Some are measures over time, others are real-time measures. Measures of academic output do not appear to capture the impact of health research in patient outcomes or practice.

7.3.7 Open Access versus Traditional Journals

Many who work in the scientific disciplines believe knowledge should be free. This is a noble purpose, and a realistic option in the digital age. OA certainly allows greater access to scientific knowledge, by switching payment structures from readers to writers. Currently, funding organizations and institutions provide funds to pay this fee, and researchers build the costs into planning and budgets. The traditional business model for publishing, where authors transfer copyright to the publisher as part of a journal agreement, is still in transition. With the emergence of OA, published knowledge is no long safely tucked away behind a pay wall, protected by the traditional subscription model. Much of this is due to the expansion of digital formats, as information is transferred and disseminated in seconds. Libraries are closing and hard copies are disappearing from racks and mailboxes. But declining subscriptions do not mean less access, as many journals are now opting for OA or hybrid formats. OA is not a philosophy, but a service and a business model (Chin 2014; Esposito 2015). It does not mean that free access is granted to everyone as soon as the work is published.

Free access is different from OA. OA refers to voluntary release of selected copyright-restricted content to the public as a marketing tool, or as a service to the profession. Editors or publishers may grant free access for periods of time at their discretion. *Public access* refers to a requirement of a funding agency stipulating that funded research results be made available to the public regardless of who holds the copyright, usually after an embargo period. Reputable publishers comply with the requirements of funding agencies to provide public access (Chin 2014).

New models and terms have created some confusion. Currently, journals are described as traditional, OA, or hybrid. Some retain subscription services and customers but offer a gold OA options for authors. OA agreements may also extend to preprints. This is a way of publishing research ahead of peer review to accelerate new knowledge. Preprints are posted online but have not been formally peer-reviewed by the scientific community, with the aim of disseminating important findings to meet an urgent need (e.g., during the COVID-19 pandemic in 2020). All forms of OA define licensing terms clearly stating how authors receive attribution and recognition for their work or any parts of that work that are reproduced.

7.3.8 Editor Query

Searching for the right journal for your research is an important step. It may lead you to find new resources and mentors. Most authors "shop around" until they find a suitable venue – one that is consistent with their personal and professional goals, or feels like the "right fit." The journal you end up selecting may not be as prestigious as your first choice, but it may be more appropriate in terms of topic and audience (Esposito 2015).

Saver (2017) recommends reading several articles from the selected journal that interest you. Review the topics and mission statement. Once selected, it is a good idea to reach out to the journal to discuss your idea or area of research. Most editors accept query letters or emails, but some do not. Instead, they ask that the author submit a cover letter with their manuscript submission. The journal website will direct this process. If query letters or communications are accepted, contact the editor directly to determine if there is an interest in your research. This step can be completed as you begin your research study, during the course of your study, or upon completion of the study. Each time frame has advantages. For the novice researcher, an early contact is preferred as the editor may be able to offer advice about methods and reporting guidelines. For example, for authors conducting a qualitative study, the editor may direct them to use specific guidelines to shape the reporting aspects of the study. This often guides the author to refine aspects of the study protocol.

Contacting the editor is a great opportunity to introduce your research or idea, and also to "sell" yourself as a worthy contributor. This step is also helpful in discussing time-sensitive matters. The editor will be interested to know if your research is complete or in progress, and will determine whether your manuscript will be a timely addition to the journal. Some journals recommend that authors submit completed works directly to them. If this is the case, the work will be committed to the journal but the journal will not execute finality to the author until the review process is complete. Often, much time is wasted if the work is rejected and the author chooses to re-submit to another journal.

Pre-submission query has many benefits. The editor can give feedback about your idea, and help direct your writing to meet the requirements of the journal. Additionally, the editor may direct your work toward a unique slant or focus that is congruent with the mission of the journal or in tangent with an upcoming issue. Conversely, the editor may inform you that the topic is not of interest to them, or is something they have in progress. Thus, they may inform you that it would be best to pursue another journal for a timelier publication. Often, they will refer you to a journal that might be a better fit for your topic. Such early communication is advantageous to the editor as it allows them to plan ahead in anticipation of the topic, schedule the topic for a special or topical issue, and work with you to ensure that the journal guidelines, IFA, and methodological guidelines used by reviewers are utilized. Additionally, they can begin to select reviewers and alert them of a pending assignment.

As you begin your communication to the editor, realize that this may be the beginning of a long and beneficial professional relationship. Identify yourself and define your project succinctly. Offer enough detail to clearly represent your work. Personalize your correspondence, addressing the letter to the editor or editorial representative identified on the journal's website. Make sure the editor has a clear idea of your work, timeline, and commitment. It is always helpful to include some information that shows your exposure to the journal. Be sure to spell-check and grammar-check your letter, as this will be an indicator of your abilities and work ethic. Sample query letters are found in most publishing texts, workbooks, and seminars.

7.4 Writing, Reviewing, and Revising

Writing is hard work. Although it is a critical communication skill, it does not come easily to everyone. It is a process of sequential steps that are quite narrowly defined for scientific purposes. Nurses have extensive expertise in clinical practice, and are well suited to informing and educating colleagues within nursing and other disciplines. Yet, the process of writing for professional publication can be daunting. It has distinct aspects in any form. One is the writing process itself, including the rules, mechanics, and flow of the work. Another is the format and requirements of the discipline, the research itself, the journal, and the publisher. Research article formats are quite prescriptive, calling for a logical, coherent structure. The writing should be clear, offering a precis and an accurate description of the study. Scientific writing has limited flexibility, often within a structured template that does not dictate the content but does direct the format (Alexander 2017).

7.4.1 Transforming Student Papers

One important distinction about scientific writing is that it is very different from writing an academic paper. Students' academic papers should never be submitted to a professional journal, but they may serve as a starting point for writing for publication. Faculty should encourage students to write. They should also explain how to transform a student paper, which demonstrates what the student knows about a subject, into a professional paper, which is written with the reader in mind, offering new knowledge or a new perspective. They should encourage students to explore journal websites in order to understand the publication process and to consider adapting their work to meet the professional standards described (Kennedy 2016). Cowell and Pierson (2016) offer an excellent writing guide for students as part of the INANE Student Papers Work Group. It is a generous resource for faculty and students as they transition to professional publication.

7.4.2 Before Writing Begins: Author Instructions, Resources, Templates, and Guidelines

Before beginning to write, search your journal of choice and become familiar with its IFA. Obtain specific reporting guidelines, designed as a checklist and flowchart, that are recommended for your research design. Together, these two resources will guide your written research report. Often, links within the IFA will guide you to specific guidelines and resources. These are a gift, adding structure and organization to the formal writing process. Additionally, your chosen journal may have editorials or articles in its archives that discuss the publishing process, offer writing tips, and review specific journal guidelines in detail.

Every research report must have logical flow. The work must be presented in an organized manner as the authors introduces the idea or aim of the study and move through each step of the research process, adding detail, explanation, and references as needed. Often, the manuscript reads like a chronology, and it should closely resemble the format used to submit the research to an institutional review board (IRB). Research formats are widely available, although they will be somewhat more structured for quantitative research (e.g., the Introduction, Methods, Results, and Discussion [IMRAD] format). Qualitative research reports follow similar but different reporting structures; there are many resources available to guide the writer.

7.4.3 Types of Publication Guidelines

7.4.3.1 Journal-Specific Guidelines

Journal and research reporting guidelines, used in combination with good writing techniques, can help authors with manuscript preparation. However, they are distinctly different tools. Journal guidelines inform the potential author about requirements that are unique to the individual journal. These may be referred to as "journal guidelines," "IFA," or simply "guidelines for authors." They are easily discovered through links on the journal website.

It is important for authors to review the journal guidelines before beginning the writing process, as this can reduce unnecessary revision and early rejections. It is unsettling to editors when they open a new submission and find that the reference style, word count, tables, and figures are not consistent with the journal instructions. In some cases, this indicates that the authors are ill informed, not detail oriented, or not selective. It may even be a "red flag" that suggest that the manuscript was submitted in a generic format and possibly submitted to other journals concurrently. If the editor does choose to move the manuscript into review, it will already be deemed to require a major revision, as these points must be addressed before the article moves forward to the peer review and revision stage. Each journal specifies its preferred style and format, but most nursing journals follow these two style guides: APA and AMA. Oermann et al. (2018b) conducted a study of 245 nursing journals and found their guidelines were easily accessible and generally complete and informative.

7.4.3.2 Guidelines for Reporting Health Research: The EQUATOR Network and Beyond

In addition to journal-specific guidelines, instructions will be available for specific types of research reporting, such as health research. Most can be accessed on the Enhancing the Quality and Transparency of Health Research (EQUATOR) network. These tools, guidelines, checklists, and templates are distributed free of charge through professional networks. EQUATOR is made up of authors, researchers, editors, and others with an interest in improving the quality of research publications. It is an international initiative that aims to improve the reliability and value of the published health research literature by distribution robust reporting guidelines specific to qualitative studies.

7.4.3.3 Qualitative Reporting Guidelines

Qualitative research typically focuses on collecting very detailed information with small sample sizes, often addresses meaning rather than objectively identifiable factors. This means that typical markers of research quality for quantitative studies, such as validity and reliability, cannot accurately assess qualitative research. However, there are many measures/tools that can be used to assess it. The first three listed by the EQUATOR network are Standards for Reporting Qualitative Research (SRQR), Consolidated Criteria for Reporting Qualitative Research (COREQ), and Enhancing Transparency in Reporting the Synthesis of Qualitative Research (ENTREQ). Others are published by the APA,

Table 7.1 Reporting guidelines for qualitative research papers.

Type of Study	Guidelines
Qualitative	SRQR: Standards for Reporting Qualitative Research (O'Brien et al. 2014)
Qualitative (focus groups and inter-views)	COREQ: COnsolidated criteria for REporting Qualitative Research (Tong et al. 2007)
Qualitative reporting standards	JARS-Qual: Journal Article Reporting Standards (American Psychological Association 2020)
Mixed methods appraisal tool	MMAT version 2018 (Hong et al. 2018)
Mixed method designs	JARS-Mixed (APA 2020)
Synthesis of qualitative research	ENTREQ: the Enhancing Transparency in Reporting the Synthesis of Qualitative Research (Tong et al. 2012).
Tools at UNC University Libraries (n.d.)	EQUATOR Network
	CASP Critical Assessment Tools for Evaluating Qualitative Research
	Joanna Briggs Institute (JBI) Tools for Qualitative Research
	Qualitative Research Review Guideline: RATS British Medical Journal
	NICE Quality Appraisal Checklist for Qualitative Studies 3rd edn.
	McMaster University Review Forms for Qualitative Studies

AMA, and professional organizations such as the Joanna Briggs Institute. Table 7.1 lists some frequently used reporting guidelines for qualitative reports. Each item on a checklist is associated with definitions and explanations of key elements, with examples to illustrate how the SRQR can be met while preserving the requisite flexibility to accommodate various paradigms, approaches, and methods.

7.5 Understanding Publishing Contracts

The journal, book, or venue selected for publication will have specific contracts that are standardized and vetted by the publisher's legal and professional staff. These are usually accessible through the journal website or communicated to the author before final agreements are complete. Additionally, many journals publish additional information to help authors navigate these agreements (Gould 2017). As this can be confusing, it is important to understand some of the standard definitions and terms of publication. Contracts and agreements are designed to fit the traditional publishing models discussed earlier in this chapter as well as OA models, including fully OA journals, hybrid journals and institutional agreements, and self-archiving or green OA.

As the author of a work, you are the exclusive copyright holder unless or until you transfer your rights. Copyright licenses detail the rights for publication, distribution, and use of research. All authors must sign a license agreement before publication. Copyright gives the author exclusive rights to reproduce, distribute, display, and prepare transitional or other derivative work, and to reuse the work in teaching, future publication, and all professional activates. Retention of copyright also allows the author to self-archive or post their work online or in an institutional repository. There are many considerations to take into account before you sign away your work. It is important to understand copyright laws and agreements.

Copyright protection exists as soon as a work is created, and may be registered through the Copyright Clearance Center or directly with the U.S. Copyright Office. It is important to know that the author does own the original work, unless it is considered work for hire in which case it belongs to the employer. Copyright may be transferred to a publisher, with some rights negotiated and retained. The Creative Commons group will help you publish your work online while letting others know exactly what they can and can't do with it. Creative Commons licenses are at the center of a major shift in how scientific research is conducted and shared, as they offer a choice for authors.

Research supported by a grant or some type of funding organization may direct the dissemination of a work. Some research funders request or require that work created with their funds be made available openly on the Web. Electronic licensing agreements are similar to traditional licensing arrangements, but the terms may define on what platform (hardware or operating systems) or in what markets the work will appear.

7.6 The Writing Process

As the writing process begins, the author should have all the tools they require at hand, including basic definitions (Paradis 2016), sample research formats from the selected journal, the journal's IFA, reporting guidelines, resources for guiding scientific writing such as APA or AMA guidelines, and resources for authors and writers (Pinker 2015; Saver 2017; Strunk and White 1959; Zinsser 2016). Many digital writing aids are available at no or little charge, which go well beyond spell checking to help authors with the writing and editing process. Grammarly and stylistic tools such as the Hemmingway Editor are widely used (Write Life 2020).

Writing is a skill that can be learned, and certainly improved upon. Like most skills, it takes practice and the rejection of learned behaviors. Prepare by identifying barriers to your writing and identifying weakness or deficits in your learning. Many publishers provide author resources that include sample manuscripts, writing tools, podcasts, online courses, and publication manuals. An example is *Editage*, a publication-focused editing service, which provides Web-based author guidance and virtual courses for authors and peer reviewers. Wolters Kluwer sponsors *Editage* in partnership with Lippincott Williams & Wilkins. Many services are offered free of charge. Even though some resources and guidelines are specific to a particular publisher, the information

Table 7.2 Writing resources.

Nurse Author and Editor Journal
International Academy of Nursing Editors (INANE)
American Journal of Nursing Writing Resources
Editage, Wolters Kluwer Writers Services
Wiley Author Services
Journal of Midwifery and Woman's Health (JMWF) Series on Writing for Publication
Writing for Professional Journals Course, Dr. Patricia Gonce Morton, University of Utah
Elsevier Publishing Campus

will be informative for authors publishing in any journal. For example, the *American Journal of Nursing* offers a series of free articles about professional writing. Roush (2017) begins this series, which helps nurses develop good writing habits and skills. It takes nurses step-by-step though the publishing process, looking at how manuscripts get published and why, how to submit an article, how to work with editors, and how to avoid common pitfalls. Frances Likis, editor of the *Journal of Midwifery and Women's Health* (JMWF), offers a series of free editorials that provide excellent guidelines addressing the submission and peer review processes, authorship, journal selection, and other advice on the publication process (Likis 2020). A list of writing resources is presented in Table 7.2.

A plethora of virtual and live formats exist to educate authors at every level. Professional organizations and universities often provide similar services. Publication workshops are offered at professional meetings, online, and through professional writing groups such as the American Association of Medical Writers. Nursing and other editors are often speakers and frequent authors on this topic. Many are available for consult at conferences sponsored by professional organizations.

7.6.1 Individual Writing Tips

Some general writing tips include the following. If you have an idea, or are beginning a research study, do not simply sit down and to write. Review the literature and resources that are readily available, and do some due diligence on the topic, journals, and current state of scholarly publication. Keep research articles from your target journal on hand, and take note of the cadence and flow of the work. Stay in contact with the editor if possible, and address concerns or questions early. Every writer must find what works for them, but you may replicate new styles and incorporate new learning from other writers, editors, and many different resources. A successful writer may apply lessons from other disciplines. Branwyn (2019) tells writers to continue to read extensively and learn new ways to express thoughts, concepts, and findings. David P. Stevens, editor-in-chief of *Quality and Safety in Health Care*, has designed a reflective exercise that may help new writers gain a better sense of their goals, challenges, and expectations, using four questions or prompts: (i) Do you find writing fun?; (ii) How frequently do you actually sit down and write for scholarly purposes?; (iii) Reflect on your experience writing scholarly papers for publication; and (iv) What do you consider your strengths in scholarly writing for health care improvement or for other purposes? (Stevens n.d.).

7.6.2 Tips for Specific Sections of the Article

The title, abstract, and introduction are the essence of your work. Be clear and parsimonious. As you craft your introduction, know that you will fully develop the background through the literature review. The literature review should be a synthesis of what is known and where gaps exist, presenting validation for the research study. As you organize your paper, use many headings, as these may become transitional headers or sentences that can help with reorganization in later stages. While writing each section, refer back to the IFA and specific qualitative research guidelines. When preparing research reports, remember to use your proposal or IRB as a guide. In the methods section, describe the ethical considerations. IRB committees and international review boards are the only bodies that can approve, exempt, or re-qualify a study.

The methods and design sections appear next. Be clear about the methods that were used. Provide sufficient detail on each. When describing the qualitative method, clearly describe the specific approach, which may be: phenomenology, grounded theory, or ethnography. Research design refers to the blueprint that you prepared using your chosen research method, and delineates the steps that you took to answer the research question. If the wrong research method or design was used, your article will be rejected by the editor no matter how well it is written (Morton 2017).

For qualitative studies, describe the data analysis and procedures used in detail. Show evidence of your meticulous attention to language and images. Describe the process of deep reflection, and how patterns and meaning emerged. Describe the processes for coding, thematic analysis, and categorization. You may use manual or electronic methods; many researchers use both. Saldana (2016) provides an excellent coding manual with a comprehensive appendix for coding methods and analytic recommendations. Support your choices with references and statements showing that you used appropriate procedures and were informed by a valid approach and methodology. Although your data may be presented in words and not in statistical charts, the data collection and reporting methods should be rigorous and appropriate for the data collected. Tables with supporting data, such as quotes to support themes, are well suited to most journal formats. Discuss the specific method of interview or focus group and why you chose it. Explain the procedures that you followed in enough detail that key elements of the methods are supported. Throughout the methods sections, be mindful of the vital "who?", "what?", "where?", "when?", and "how?" questions of qualitative research (Cypress 2015). Researchers from all disciplines use these approaches according to the purpose of their study. A clear explanation that links the purpose and approach is necessary. Each approach requires sufficient description, including aspects of data analysis and citations in its support. The authors' job is to describe which approach guided the study, through data collection and analysis.

The discussion section is best organized by the research question, and builds support for the conclusion. Here is where many authors "run out of gas," but it is important to include details with clearly stated limitations and recommendations, including lessons learned (Morton 2017). Finally, the conclusion "wraps up" the study. This is another area that is often lacking, as authors hurry to end the long hours of research and writing. However, it is a section that can be rich with innovations and ideas for future research.

An important concept in writing, in the conclusion and throughout the paper, is "voice." The reader should be able to recognize the voice of the writer. Too often, readers wish the writer's voice had come through. Editors may request that an author extends their work to expand their voice. Your writing may be formal, factual, and important to the scientific process, but voice has a place in the message. Tell the audience why this is important to you, to the practice, to the patients. Share what you have learned and suggest how the reader may use your work (Gould 2019).

7.6.3 Combating Procrastination, Defeat, Exhaustion, and Other Real-Life Responsibilities

Time management is always an essential part of writing. It reflects a personal awareness of what barriers and support systems work for each individual. Identify "time wasters," procrastinating behaviors, and other barriers that are known obstacles. Be realistic about deadlines and work with your writing time, adjusting to ensure success. Editors and colleagues know that things happen. Responsibilities change, children and family needs shift, and often things occur outside of anyone's control – such as in 2020, when a global pandemic changed everything. Choose a location and time that support personal writing habits, and realize that these may require change. During the pandemic, home became a writer's sanctuary for some and a source of tremendous stress for others. Office spaces closed and workflow changed dramatically.

7.6.4 Things to Remember Before You Submit Your Manuscript

Editors have little tolerance for sloppy work. Be mindful of the writing steps, use guidelines, and spend time on editing. Read and listen to experts. Don't confuse writing and revising. They require two very different approaches. Writing may flow best without complex rules, but revisions are guided by rules and distinctions put forth by the publication (Gould 2019). Many revisions may be required before the work can be submitted to the journal. This is part of the process, and it is often said that the work of writing is truly visible in the revisions. Friends, colleagues, and relatives may serve as readers. Often, authors will employ editing services prior to submitting. It is important to alert all readers and personal reviewers about specific guidelines that are required by the selected journal.

7.7 Submitting the Manuscript

First, create a password-protected account on the publisher's site. This serves for both author and reviewer services. Become proficient with the publishing software, as it the vehicle for all communication, including author agreements, submission, permissions, peer review, revisions, copyediting, and final proofs. These are linked directly from the journal website. After submission, you will be able to digitally track your manuscript and see when it has moved through technical checks, editor assignment, and peer review. The editor-in-chief or assigned editor will communicate about acceptance, revisions, and rejections.

As you submit the final manuscript, be mindful of specific instructions regarding loading files and author identification. Title and author pages are usually loaded as individual files. This allows the production team to blind authors names and other identifiers for peer review. Tables, figures, permissions and other documents are loaded as separate files or follow the manuscript.

7.8 The Peer Review Process

Peer review is the structure that defines scholarly work. Saver (2017) reminds us that publishing is a team sport. The authors provide the raw materials, often guided by editorial guidelines and professional traditions. Peer review is then the critical assessment of manuscripts submitted to journals by experts who are usually not part of the editorial staff. The International Committee of Medical Journal Editors (ICMJE 2019) describes peer review as an important extension of the scientific process and the defining step in scholarly publication. The peer review process is a two-way street. Writers often serve as peer reviewers and expert consultants for journals. Expert reviewers provide content knowledge and expertise to give a "fair hearing" to a manuscript. They offer questions, comments, and suggestions, which always strengthen the work and help editors determine if it should be rejected or accepted, with minor or major revisions. Peer reviewers serve as content advisors and may review research protocols, re-evaluate data, or serve as developmental editors, if needed. Editors include peer reviewers in communication about rejection, revision, and acceptance. This includes the comments from all reviewers, as well as authors' responses to reviewers' comments. As authors revise and resubmit, reviewers can read the authors' responses, including detailed replies or rebuttals for each reviewer comment. This is a tremendous learning opportunity for the peer reviewer.

7.8.1 After Peer Review: A Decision

If a paper is considered for publication, it will be classified as reject, revise, or resubmit, with caveats for minor or major revisions, and an indication of whether it will be sent for re-review. Reviewers often provide detailed comments. These may be attached in the form of a list or table or added directly to the manuscript using track-editing tools. Reviewer comments always serve to make the manuscript stronger. Authors are asked to respond to all of the comments in detail, providing a reply in the form of a revision, rebuttal, or clarification. Reviewer comments are included even when a rejection is determined. The editor may add some additional comments directing the author to other journals or explaining in more detail why the manuscript was rejected. Often, this communication is a valuable tool to help the author revise the manuscript for submission in another journal.

7.8.2 Revisions and Resubmitting

Although a decision to revise is not an acceptance, and completing a revision will not guarantee acceptance, revision is an important step toward seeing your work in print. A manuscript will be rated as requiring major or minor revision. Do not be discouraged, as what may appear to be a major revision might be quite easy following the detailed instructors of the peer review team and editor. This is a small hurdle to cross, as the research and most of the writing is done!

It is important to remember that the critique is not personal. It is meant to improve the manuscript and move it toward publication for the selected journal. Be flexible and allow change to become a part of what you do. If something is not working and you cannot change, then you cannot improve. Use lessons from *improvement science*, which works for everything – even writing. Improvement work reminds us that doing the same thing and expecting different results simply does not work. Revisions may require that you cut words, phrases, or sections to provide a more parsimonious article. As an editor and a "prepositional phrase abuser," I target this first. I recently became aware that I use adverbs to the exclusion of the verb. If I cannot see this myself, I use writing apps such as Hemmingway Editor. Although I do not edit with the rigor the app suggests, I find sentences are crisper and clearer.

As you revise, remember that this is an opportunity to strengthen your work – a gift from experts and professional you may never have the chance to meet in person.

Use many tools, mentors, readers, and professional resources. Contact the editor with specific questions. Even in a digital world, there are opportunities for phone calls, Zoom meeting, and private emails. An offer to revise is a chance to succeed. There are excellent resources available to help guide your revision. Pierson (2016) offers advice for revision and resubmission, covering the important steps of read, reflect, revise and rewrite, and respond.

7.9 The Production Process

Accepted manuscripts must go through many additional steps before online and print publication becomes a reality. Publishers have production teams that provide technical and professional services at many levels, including copyediting, formatting, reference checking, permissions checking, and journal set-up (e.g., staging and page assignment). Spelling and grammar checks, mathematical validation, statistical tables, reference checks, funding validation, and crosscheck all continue up to final production. Some journals add additional scientific editing by subject matter experts. Upon acceptance, the manuscript will be assigned to a member of the production team, who will oversee this work with the editor and author toward final publication. The author will see and approve the final proofs and respond to editorial queries before the final work is set up within the issue.

7.9.1 Working With Your Editor

As a group, editors are knowledgeable and generous professionals. Their goal is to move science forward though scholarly work. It is important that you have access to and guidance from your editor through emails and other forms of agreed-upon communication. Freda and Nicoll (2011) provide a handbook for editors, sharing advice and techniques that can help them improve in their profession. An excellent writer's blog, *The Scholarly Kitchen*, offers many insights into the work of editors and advice for working with them (Anderson 2013).

7.9.2 How Editors and Publishers Make Decisions

Editors plan and organize each issue and determine the overall direction of the journal. They are usually content experts, have advanced education, and are guided by publishers and professional regulatory and advisory groups such as COPE and the ICMJE, and by professional writing organizations such as the American Medical Writers Associations (AMWA). Editors-in-chief hold broad authority and have significant editorial freedom, as defined by the ICMJE (2019). Advice from editors takes many forms, often defined within the journal's IFA, editorials, and other written works. Nurse authors, editors, publishers, and professional organizations continue to inform nurse writers and editors.

7.10 Dissemination and Marketing

Dissemination is a long but rewarding process. Gennaro (2018) reminds researchers that conducting and writing up excellent research is only the first step. You must also help others find your science. Techniques such as search engine optimization (SEO), publication in high-quality journals that are indexed in major databases, and social media presence (including tweeting about your research) will aid others in discovering your writing. Work with your publisher to disseminate your work in other formats. Most journals will submit press releases for you, and provide letters to employers, tenure committees, and others as requested. Many offer PowerPoint slides of all tables and figures that appear in your article, with citation and attribution for the author and publisher. Editors may assist in preparing promotional slides for presentations or recognition events. They will always give you an opportunity to respond to letters to the editor, and will often publish your reply concurrently. Many publishers provide a free pdf of the article upon publication, with clear guidelines for reuse and distribution.

7.11 Conclusion

Quality is everything. Every author wants to produce something that they are proud of and which will inform, inspire, and lead current practice and future generations. As new and experienced authors continue to write, present, and share knowledge, the resources and information within this chapter reflect the work of many nurse authors, editors, scientists, and scholars who write well and write often. It is with sincere gratitude that we share and acknowledge the work of all the people referenced in this chapter.

References

Albert, T. and Wagner, E. (2003). How to handle authorship disputes: a guide for new researchers. The COPE Report. Available from https://publicationethics.org/files/2003pdf12_0.pdf (accessed May 10, 2021).

Alexander, M. (2017). Organizing the article. In: Anatomy of Writing for Publication, 3e (ed. C. Savor), 68–78. Sigma Theta Tau International.

American Psychological Association (2020). Journal article reporting standards. Reporting standards for qualitative research. In: Publication Manual of the American Psychological Association, 7c, 101. American Psychological Association.

Anderson, K. (2013). Updated – 73 things publishers do (2013 edition). The Scholarly Kitchen. Available from https://scholarlykitchen.sspnet.org/2013/10/22/updated-73-things-publishers-do-2013-edition (accessed May 10, 2021).

Branwyn G. (2019). How to be a better writer: tips, tricks, and hard-won lessons: from creating drafts to working with editors. Medium. May 29. Available from https://medium.com/better-humans/how-to-be-abetter-writer-a3c877f67a5c (accessed May 10, 2021).

Chin, P. (2014). Open access: what it is and what it is not. Advances in Nursing Science Blog. November 26. Available from https://ansjournalblog.com/2014/11/26/open-access-what-it-is-and-what-it-is-not/ (accessed May 10, 2021).

COPE. (2018). How to recognize potential authorship problems. Available from https://publicationethics.org/resources/flowcharts/how-recognise-potential-authorship-problems (accessed May 10, 2021).

COPE (2021). Update on COPE guidance regarding author name changes. COPE Digest 9 (1).

Cowell, J.M. and Pierson, C. (2016). Helping students get published: tips from journal editors. A white paper developed by the INANE Student Papers Work Group. Nurse Author Editor 26 (4): 6.

Cypress, B. (2015). Qualitative research: the "what," "why," and "how"! Dimensions of Critical Care Nursing 34 (6): 356–361.

Cypress, B. (2017). Exploring the philosophical, paradigmatic, conceptual-theoretical underpinnings of qualitative research: a focus on a phenomenological study in intensive care unit. Dimensions of Critical Care Nursing 36 (3): 208–216.

Cypress, B. (2018). Qualitative research methods: a phenomenological focus. Dimensions of Critical Care Nursing 37 (6): 302–309.

Cypress, B. (2020). Effective mentoring relationships in qualitative research. Dimensions of Critical Care Nursing 39 (6): 305–311.

Esposito, J. (2015). Making a case for open access. The Scholarly Kitchen. Available from http://scholarlykitchen.sspnet.org/2015/01/05/making-a-case-for-open-access/?utm_source=feedburner&utm_medium=email&utm_campaign=Feed%3A+ScholarlyKitchen+%28The+Scholarly+Kitchen%29 (accessed May 10, 2021).

Freda, M.C. and Nicoll, L.H. (2011). The Editor's Handbook: An Online Resource and CE Course. Lippincott Williams & Wilkins.

Gennaro, S. (2018). How can we disseminate nursing science more effectively? Journal of Nursing Scholarship 50 (2): 111–112.

Gould, K.A. (2017). Tips for submitting a manuscript to DCCN. Dimensions of Critical Care Nursing 36 (2): 140–141.

Gould, K.A. (2019). Writing for publication: expanding professional practice. Dimensions of Critical Care Nursing 38 (5): 233–235.

Hein, L.C. and Chin, P. (2017). Issues of authorship: who and in what order? Nurse Author and Editor 27 (3): 6.

Hong, Q., Gonzalez-Reyes, A., and Pluye, P. (2018). Improving the usefulness of a tool for appraising the quality of qualitative, quantitative, and mixed methods studies, the Mixed Methods Appraisal Tool (MMAT). Journal of Evaluation in Clinical Practice 24: 459–467.

ICMJE. (2019). Recommendations for the conduct, reporting, editing and publication of scholarly work in medical journals. Available from http://www.icmje.org/icmje-recommendations.pdf (accessed May 10, 2021).

ICMJE. (2021) Roles and responsibilities of authors, contributors, reviewers, editors, publishers, and owners. Available from http://www.icmje.org/recommendations/browse/roles-and-responsibilities (accessed May 10, 2021).

INANE. (n.d.). Airtable – nursing journal directory. Available from https://airtable.com/shrjqveaKHtS9xku8/tblNXTxmTr18CC1If (accessed May 10, 2021).

Kennedy, M.S. (2016). My professor said to submit my paper: we hope they also told you this. Dimensions of Critical Care Nursing 35 (1): 23–24.

Likis, F. (2020). Writing for publication [editorials]. From the Journal of Midwifery and Women's Health (JMWF). Available from https://onlinelibrary.wiley.com/doi/toc/10.1111/(ISSN)1542-2011.writingforpublication (accessed May 10, 2021).

Morton, P.G. (2017). Strategies for writing a research article: an editor's perspective. Nurse Author & Editor 27 (1): 5.

O'Brien, B.C., Harris, L., Beckman, T. et al. (2014). Standards for reporting qualitative research: a synthesis of recommendations. Academic Medicine 89 (9): 12245–12125.

Oermann, M.H. and Hays, J. (2016). Writing for Publication in Nursing, 3e. Springer.

Oermann, M.H., Nicoll, L.H., Chinn, P.L. et al. (2018a). Quality of articles published in predatory nursing journals. Nursing Outlook 66 (1): 4–10.

Oermann, M.H., Nicoll, L.H., Chinn, P.L. et al. (2018b). Quality of author guidelines in nursing journals. Journal of Nursing Scholarship 50 (3): 333–340.

Paradis, E. (2016). The tools of the qualitative research trade. Academic Medicine 91 (12): e17.

Pierson, C. (2016). The four R's of revising and resubmitting a manuscript. Journal of the American Association of Nurse Practitioners 28: 408–409.

Pinker, S. (2015). The Sense of Style: The Thinking person's Guide to Writing in the 21st Century. Penguin Books.

Polit, D.F. and Beck, C.T. (2021). Nursing Research: Generating and Assessing Evidence for Nursing Practice, 11e. Wolters Kluwer.

Roush, K. (2017). Becoming a published writer. American Journal of Nursing 117 (3): 63–66.

Saldana, J. (2016). The Coding Manual for Qualitative Research. Sage Publications.

Sandelowski, M. (1995). Sample size in qualitative research. Research in Nursing and Health 18 (2): 179–183.

Saver, C. (2017). Anatomy of Writing for Publication, 3e. Sigma Theta Tau International.

Stevens, D. (n.d.) Guided reflection on your writing. Institute for Healthcare Improvement. Available from http://www.ihi.org/education/IHIOpenSchool/resources/Pages/Publications/GuidedReflectionOnYourWriting.aspx (accessed May 10, 2021).

Strunk, W. and White, E.B. (1959). The Elements of Style. Macmillan.

Tong, A., Sainsbury, P., and Craig, J. (2007). Consolidated criteria for reporting qualitative research (COREQ): a 32-item checklist for interviews and focus groups. International Journal for Quality in Health Care 19 (6): 349–357.

Tong, A., Flemming, K., McInnis, E. et al. (2012). Enhancing transparency in Reporting the synthesis of qualitative research: ENTREQ. BMJ Medical Research Methodology 12: 181.

UNC University Libraries. (n.d.). Qualitative research resources. Available from https://guides.lib.unc.edu/qual/assess (accessed May 10, 2021).

Write Life. (2020). Six grammar checkers and editing tools to make your writing super clean. Updated January 20. Available from https://thewritelife.com/automatic-editing-tools (accessed May 10, 2021).

Zinsser, W. (2016). On Writing Well: The Classic Guide to Writing Nonfiction. Harper Perennial.

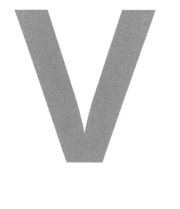

V Practical Aspects of Qualitative Phenomen- ological Research

8

Challenges and Dilemmas in Phases of Qualitative Research

I have been conducting, teaching, and writing about qualitative research for a number of years. There are many different stories that research students and novices can tell about their experiences of the challenges and dilemmas that arise before, during, and after the laborious process of carrying out a naturalistic inquiry. I do not pretend that these testimonies are typical, for investigators encounter varied circumstances unique to their studies. There are also a myriad of suggestions and pointers present in the literature on how to address the quandaries of these investigations. It helps to revisit and make familiar to early researchers the hurdles and issues related to qualitative studies. The purpose of this chapter is to teach the skills of qualitative research in the context of the practical problems that doctoral students and beginners face in different phases of the endeavor, namely: selecting a topic, exploring the literature, selecting the setting, considering ethical perspectives, choosing a methodology and research design, and collecting, managing, and analyzing data.

8.1 Conceptualizing and Starting a New Qualitative Study

8.1.1 Selecting a Topic

Qualitative research is conducted when little is known about a phenomenon or when present knowledge or theories about it may be biased. The researcher aims to develop a rich and context-bound understanding of the poorly-understood phenomenon in a naturalistic setting (Morse and Field 1995; Polit and Beck 2017). Thinking about, defining, and deciding what phenomenon to study is the hardest step of a qualitative research endeavor (Neiswiadomy and Bailey 2018). Research problems do not arise out of a clear blue sky (Silverman 2005)! This is usually the first challenge encountered by novices and new researchers. Many doctoral students become "lost" in this first step, resulting in a long and agonizing journey toward completing their dissertation or first naturalistic inquiry. How should a new researcher decide on a topic? What phenomena important to nursing lend themselves to a qualitative inquiry?

Fundamentals of Qualitative Phenomenological Nursing Research, First Edition. Brigitte S. Cypress.
© 2022 John Wiley & Sons Ltd. Published 2022 by John Wiley & Sons Ltd.

Research is a time-consuming enterprise, so curiosity about and interest in a topic are essential to a project's success (Polit and Beck 2017). Selecting a research topic to study through qualitative methods is a very risky activity. It involves committing oneself to a particular course of action rather than reiterating "spoon-fed" critiques (Silverman 2005). At the most basic level, research topics originate with the investigator's interests. Morse and Field (1995) encourage questions such as, "What articles catch my eye when I am in the library?" and, "What topics do I constantly think about and often discuss in general conversations?" (p. 45). There are other explicit sources that can help in finding a study topic, and eventually a phenomenon: one might consider significant experiences that have occurred in clinical practice, an observation that is not documented in the literature, or gaps in patient-care literature recommendations and actual practice (Morse and Field 1995). Ideas can also come from gaps in the nursing literature in general, from global social or political issues like health disparities, or from external sources like funding agencies' research priorities (Polit and Beck 2014). At times, investigators who already have a program of research may get inspiration from their own findings. Morse and Field (1995) note that:

> Finding a topic takes some self-examination, and discussing one's ideas with colleagues and experienced qualitative researchers is essential. The researcher must find the topic chosen to be fascinating because working 6 months on a boring topic convert what should be an exciting activity into drudgery. (p. 45)

Once a topic is decided on, it is important to identify and try to state the phenomenon and to pose a research question. Table 8.1 presents examples of phenomena and research questions from previously conducted qualitative studies.

Table 8.1 Phenomena and research questions in qualitative studies.

1. What are the lived experiences of newly qualified nurses on clinical placement during the first six months following registration in the Republic of Ireland? (O'Shea and Kelly 2007)
2. What are the nurses' experiences of recruitment and migration from developing countries? (Troy et al. 2007)
3. What are the experiences of homeless people in the healthcare delivery system? (Martins 2008)
4. What are nursing students' lived experiences of empowerment and being valued? (Bradbury-Jones et al. 2011)
5. What are nurses' experiences with nursing research and its integration in practice? (Dupin et al. 2012)

8.1.2 Exploring the Literature

Opinions about literature review in qualitative research vary. For example, no literature review is done in a grounded theory study (Glaser 1978; Morse and Field 1995; Polit and Beck 2017): the researcher typically begins to collect the data before searching what is in the literature. Phenomenologists and ethnographers, on the other hand, do undertake a preliminary review at the outset of a study: phenomenological studies do not require a thorough literature search, but ethnographic research needs some familiarity with what is out there to help the investigators shape their ideas about a cultural problem before entering the field (Polit and Beck 2014). Questions usually asked are: "What is the current evidence on this research problem?", "What do you have to say critically about what is already known?," and "Where will you find what you need to read?"

A researcher has to be prepared before embarking on a literature search about a phenomenon at hand. Some issues to think about are: (i) What disciplines relate to my topic?; (ii) How can I focus my topic to make my search more precise?; (iii) What are the main indices and abstracts relevant to my topic?; and (iv) What means of recording will be most efficient for many of the tasks I must undertake (e.g., cross-referencing)? (Silverman 2005).

Knowing where to find the literature is the second aspect to consider. There are many potential sources of information, but online searches and databases are the ones that most often present challenges to the novice investigator. A new researcher can find themselves in a labyrinth, facing endless articles and studies. Alternatively, they may get no "hits" when searching on a topic. Familiarity with computer searches and good skimming/reading skills are needed. It helps to know which databases to check, what keywords to use, and how to "fillet" publications according to your own agenda and criteria (Silverman 2005). Another challenge is in how to stay focused and maintain a critical perspective in doing a review. How much literature should be searched, and how far? Aside from knowing what to look for, one should remember that the goal of a thorough literature search and review is to appreciate and advance one's knowledge by keeping in mind the questions that need to be answered.

A common doctoral student's research trajectory aims for a completed literature review during or at the end of the first year. Programs at this point expect that the student should have a good idea of relevant work carried out by others, but it will be necessary to keep up with the new literature throughout the process so that the latest developments on the topic are taken into account (Silverman 2005). In qualitative research, however, completing and writing up a thorough literature survey in a year can mean a lot of wasted effort. Until the data analysis has been completed, no one can be certain what of the literature is relevant. It is thus recommended that the bulk of the literature reading be done around the data collection and analysis (Silverman 2005).

8.1.3 Selecting a Setting and "Getting In"

Qualitative researchers usually collect data in real-world, naturalistic settings like hospitals, homes, or the community. Obtaining access to the field site is at times not easy. Research settings can be closed or open, private or public. Closed settings are controlled by gatekeepers. Access to open settings may be freely available, but it is not always without difficulty, whether practical or ethical. For example, should the researcher intrude upon vulnerable minorities or groups, or freely access public records?

Depending on the phenomenon at hand or the research problem and the contingencies of the setting, access can be overt or covert. Data collection needs to be as overt as possible. In overt access, the impression the investigator gives is very important. There are always concerns about what kind of person the researcher is; this can be more important than the nature of the study itself. The organization or group under investigation will gauge whether the investigator can be trusted, and perhaps how easily they can be exploited and manipulated. "Getting in" involves gaining, building, and maintaining trust with the participants and the institution (Morse and Field 1995). Naturalistic inquirers should avoid giving impressions that might pose an obstacle to access and try to positively convey a perception that is appropriate to the situation. Being nonjudgmental is often key to acceptance in many settings, including subcultures other than the investigator's own (Silverman 2005). It is also critical to learn about power structures, politics, and conflicts within an institution and to demonstrate political, institutional, and personal neutrality (Morse and Field 1995).

8.1.4 Ethical Dilemmas

Qualitative researchers prefer to get close to the people and situations they are studying (Silverman 2005). When looking at people's behaviors and perceptions, or asking questions, it is important to keep in mind the values not only of the inquirer but also of the participants. From Mason (1996), Silverman (2005) discusses two ways in which ethical issues impinge upon the naturalistic investigator: (i) the rich and detailed character of qualitative research can mean intimate engagement with the public and private lives of individuals; and (ii) the changing directions and access during a qualitative study mean that new and unexpected dilemmas are likely to arise across its course (p. 258). To clarify and address these problems, investigators should be clear about what the purpose of their research is, examine which individuals or groups might be interested or affected by it, and consider the implications of the research for these parties. Consulting ethical guidelines to clarify procedures is paramount, and the informed consent form should explicitly state the intention and detailed process of the investigation. Qualitative studies require repeated contact with participants, and the research design evolves as data are gathered, so it is difficult to fully assess all risks and obtain meaningful informed consent at the outset. Consent may be an ongoing process, and is continuously negotiated. This is called "process consent."

Confidentiality and anonymity are other challenges encountered in qualitative research. Confidentiality is salient in naturalistic studies due to their in-depth nature, and anonymity is rarely possible (Polit and Beck 2017). This does not necessarily preclude intrusion, as anonymity by itself is not enough to protect a person's privacy or prevent disclosure of personal issues. Enquirers should refrain from soliciting private information that is not closely related to the research question (Mason 1996). It is also difficult for investigators to adequately disguise participants in their reports. Qualitative researchers must take extra precautions to safeguard participants' identities and prevent breaches of their confidentiality. There are several effective strategies for protecting personal information, including using secure data storage methods, removing identifier components, altering biographical details, and using pseudonyms (for individuals, places, and organizations) (Mason 1996). It is also a good idea to offer debriefing sessions to allow participants to ask questions and voice complaints. Offering participants and organizations feedback is beneficial. Referrals should be made to appropriate health, social, or psychological services as the need arises. The rights of special vulnerable groups may also need extra protection.

Vulnerable populations are at times incapable of giving fully informed consent, or may be at high risk for unintended side effects of a study. Examples are children, mentally or emotionally disabled people, severely or critically ill or physically impaired people, the terminally ill, those who are institutionalized, prisoners, and pregnant women. Researchers should pay particular attention to the ethical dimensions of their study among these groups. Their proposal will usually be subjected to external review and referred to the relevant institutional review board (**IRB**). Protective considerations for vulnerable populations should be explicitly stated in the IRB proposal or protocol. When highly sensitive issues are involved, children and other vulnerable individuals should have access to an advocate, who should be present during the initial phases of the study and ideally during data-gathering sessions (Mason 1996).

8.1.5 Choosing a Methodology and Research Design

Methodology is a general approach to studying research topics (Silverman 2005). One of the common mistakes of doctoral students and novices is choosing a methodology (quantitative versus qualitative) before their research topic or phenomenon is clearly established. A well-delineated phenomenon and an appropriately-posed research question imply a suitable methodology. As Miles and Huberman (1984) put it, "Knowing what you want to find out leads inexorably to the question of how you will get that information" (p. 42). The research should be driven by the research question, and an appropriate methodology should be selected accordingly (Morse and Field 1995). If a study's aim is to gain a deeper understanding of a "poorly understood" phenomenon that is not amenable to measurement and quantification, then a qualitative research methodology is the appropriate choice. Naturalistic inquirers should always keep in mind that qualitative research usually answers questions pertaining to "what an experience is like." This provides the reader with understanding and enables others to make sense of reality (Morse and Field 1995). There are some questions that need to be answered before deciding whether or not to use a qualitative methodology, as presented in Table 8.2.

The researcher should selectively and correctly choose an approach according to the nature of the problem and what is known about the phenomenon to be studied. Other factors, such as the maturity of the concept, the constraints of the setting, and the researcher's ability and agenda, should also be considered (Morse and Field 1995).

According to Morse and Field (1995), poor choice of methodology can threaten the validity of an investigation and may result in loss of generalizability and increased costs. They further state:

> Perhaps the most common problem in the inappropriate use of method is using inductive research design and qualitative methods when a considerable amount is known about the topic. Alternatively, it is equally invalid to use deductive research design and quantitative methods when too little is known about the topic. In the first case, researchers develop a conceptual framework and then analyze qualitative data according to the categories in the framework rather than derive the categories inductively from the data . . . A researcher who knows enough about the topic to be able to create a conceptual framework and identify variables should be using quantitative methods. (p. 15)

Table 8.2 Questions to ask regarding whether to use qualitative research.

1. What exactly am I trying to find out or understand?
2. What kind of focus on my topic do I want to achieve? Do I want to study a phenomenon or a situation in detail? Or am I mainly interested in making standardized and systematic comparisons and in accounting for variance? Does the phenomenon lend itself to study by qualitative methodology?
3. How have other researchers dealt with this topic? To what extent do I wish to align my study with this literature?
4. What practical considerations should sway my choice? How long might my study take? Do I have resources to study it this way? Can I get access to the participants I want to use? Will my planned population be accessible and available?
5. Will we learn more about this topic using a qualitative methodology? What will be the knowledge payoff in choosing this methodology?
6. What seems to work best for me? Am I committed to a particular research model which implies a particular research methodology? Do I have a gut feeling about what a good piece of research looks like?

Source: Silverman, D. (2005). *Doing Qualitative Research*, 2nd ed., Sage Publications.

Novice researchers may have some confusion about the role of theory in both quantitative and qualitative research. Theories guide both methodologies at different stages in the study process. In inductive (qualitative) research, the investigator examines the data for patterns and relationships, develops and tests hypotheses to generate a theory, or uses developed theories to explain the data. In deductive (quantitative) research, the investigator tests a developed theory (Morse and Field 1995).Although the goal of qualitative research is to develop a theory, not all qualitative research will have a theory as its end-product. A grounded theory design specifically aims to develop a mid-range theory that describes a process as its final product. This is one approach in which the research is inductively driven, although both induction and deduction are used to develop the theory.

Given that a particular phenomenon is best studied using a qualitative methodology, how should a naturalistic inquirer select the "best" or most appropriate research design? The answer will depend on the qualifications of the researcher, what they wish to know, the expected outcomes of the research, the constraints of the setting, the participants, and the resources available (Morse and Field 1995). Theory is almost always present and embedded in qualitative research traditions (Polit and Beck 2017). A conceptualization of a specific phenomenon under study is called "substantive theory," as per Sandelowski (1993). Phenomenologists are committed to a theoretical naivety, and try to hold preconceived views of the phenomenon of interest in check, but are guided by a framework that focuses their inquiry on certain aspects of a person's lifeworld (i.e., lived experiences). Ethnographers, on the other hand, bring a cultural perspective to their studies, which helps shape their fieldwork. Ethnography is done if the purpose of the research is to describe a setting or a community. If the aim is to describe the types of healthcare professionals in that community, then ethnoscience is a more suitable approach (Morse and Field 1995). Ideational and materialistic theories are two examples of cultural theories that adopted in ethnographic investigations (Polit and Beck 2017). Phenomenology, ethnography, grounded theory, and ethnoscience are all examples of qualitative research designs. Each answers different questions, has distinct methods, and provides different perspectives on the phenomenon of interest (Morse and Field 1995). There is an appropriate research design for every question, and selecting the right one is the most important decision in the research process (Morse and Field 1995).

8.1.6 Collecting, Managing, and Analyzing Data

Qualitative research introduces moral and ethical problems during data collection and analysis. The principal investigator is the "sole instrument" of the study, being trained and fully responsible to gather and analyze the data. It is difficult to use research assistants to conduct unstructured interviews and assist with data analysis (Morse and Field 1995). Novices as interviewers may lack confidence and experience in starting, conducting, and maintaining a comfortable and fruitful interaction, including dealing with "sensitive topics" and the complex tasks of analyzing and interpreting data. Over time, the effectiveness and efficiency of data collection varies. Morse and Field (1995) suggest that fieldwork has different stages. Initially, data collection is inefficient and unfocused because researcher comprehension is low and there is accompanying confusion and bewilderment. Credibility as a researcher has to be established within the setting, including acquiring the skills of being present, trusted, and neutral. The naturalistic inquirer must fit into the setting. Selection of dress and observation of etiquette (e.g., addressing participants in the correct way) may influence one's acceptance. How one presents oneself to participants or groups may be crucial to obtaining quality data (Morse and Field 1995). Other issues can arise related to human subject participation, such as lack of willingness and rapport, concerns about confidentiality and privacy, and difficulty in interview.

Qualitative interviews are unstructured and intimate in nature, such that participants may share information not pertaining to the phenomenon under study. They may verbalize allegations or complaints about staff or services, unwanted negative behaviors and attitudes, unethical or illegal conduct, and social injustices. Simply put, they may verbalize things they never intended to tell, and interviews can thus become a "confession" (Patton 2015). From the investigator's perspective, data collection can become a time of intense emotional strain, resulting in total preoccupation with the research process and subsequent lack of sleep (Morse and Field 1995). The researcher has the responsibility to pace data collection carefully, follow professional standards, protect privileged information, and know when to keep silent and when to report. Development of personal relationships with participants may be inevitable while collecting certain data. Therefore, inquirers should seriously consider the potential impact they may have on the participants, and vice versa (Mason 1996). It is important not to get too close to participants or to "suffer" with them. Such involvement may result in the researcher's not being able to view the data analytically, and thus affect the research process.

Qualitative researchers should consider the amount of "distance" they have from the setting. Generally, nurses should not conduct studies in the unit in which they work. This can cause confusion over their role as employee versus that as researcher, leading to misunderstandings and possible violations of privacy and confidentiality. According to Morse and Field (1995), of greatest concern is that data analysis may be impeded by an investigator's familiarity with their setting. Nurses might not record data on some behavior, for example, because it is normative, and therefore beyond their awareness. If the naturalistic inquirer has no choice but to collect data in the work setting, precautions must be observed. Be aware of role conflict. Let the staff and patients know when you are in your researcher versus your staff role. Consider strategies for emotional distancing if the research topic or participants have the potential to be emotionally challenging. Always be aware of the phenomenon, and of the purpose of the study. Avoid topics that may cause discomfort among participants. Sanjari et al. (2014) state:

> Researchers should always be aware of the precise reason for involvement in a study in order to prevent undesirable personal issues. The probability of exposure to vicarious trauma as a result of the interviews needs to be evaluated. Interviewers should be properly scheduled to provide the researcher with sufficient recovery time and reduce the risk of emotional exhaustion, while allowing ample time for analysis of the objective and emotional aspects of the research. It is also necessary for the researcher to be familiar with signs of extreme fatigue and be prepared to take necessary measures before too much harm is done. (p. 4)

Most importantly, researchers should listen to and learn the language and values of the group under study. Notes should be made on everything, even if it does not appear useful and relevant, so that a more accurate picture of the context of research can be obtained. No feedback should be given to staff until the research is completed, and field notes should not be shared (Morse and Field 1995).

The challenge of qualitative analysis is to transform data into findings. No formula exists for such transformation. Direction and guidance are available, but the final destination remains unique for each inquirer, known only when – and if – it is reached (Patton 2015). Before themes can be illuminated, the first dilemma encountered is how to make sense of the massive amounts of data collected, or to "Get a sense of the whole." Doctoral students and novice researchers face the difficult task of reducing the volume of raw information, sifting the trivial from the significant, identifying patterns, and constructing a framework for communicating the essence of what the data reveal (Patton 2015). There is no significance test to run that determines whether a finding is worthy of attention, and no way of perfectly replicating an inquirer's analytical thought processes. The best advice is for the investigator equipped with their full intellect to do their best to fairly represent the data and communicate what they reveal given the purpose of the study. Qualitative inquiry depends, at every stage, on the skills, training, insights, and capabilities of the investigator (Patton 2015).

One barrier to credible qualitative findings stems from the suspicion that an analyst has shaped results according to their own predispositions and biases. A possible strategy to avoid this involves discussing predispositions and making biases explicit, to the extent possible. In phenomenological studies, for example, inquirers engage in *epoche* or bracketing.

8.2 Combating Dilemmas and the Importance of a Mentor

An effective qualitative research project can be undertaken on the basis of "keeping it simple," adhering to the methodological steps but at the same time being reasonably flexible, and addressing issues that arise before and during the process. Patton (2015) presents suggestions for graduate students considering a qualitative dissertation based on responses gathered from different people. These recommendations are discussed here. First, it is important to find an adviser and mentor who will support you in embarking on the tough long haul or journey of completing a dissertation. Even some starting qualitative researchers need an expert researcher mentor to guide and support them. Joining a support group will also help. Being with peers that are "in the same boat" as you will allow you to talk about your research together on a regular basis, share knowledge and brainstorm, problem solve, and partake in one another's successes, thus lessening the stress. Prepare to be changed. Looking deeply at other people's lives will force you to look deeply at yourself. Be sure that you're prepared to deal with the controversies of doing qualitative research. Understand the paradigms and politics. Researchers should not elect to use qualitative methodology because they feel that it is easier (this is a misconception!); rather, they should keep in mind that there is an appropriate approach for every research problem or phenomenon. Do it because you want to, and are convinced that it is right for you. Qualitative research is time-consuming, intimate, and intense. You will need to find your questions interesting if you want to remain "sane" during the process, and at the end. Be sure that a qualitative design fits the research question. Study qualitative inquiry. There are lots of different approaches, and there is a lot to know. Learn and know methodology and design. Qualitative designs follow a different logic from quantitative ones. Practice interviewing and observation skills. Do lots of interviews. Spend a lot of time doing practice fieldwork observations. Get feedback from someone who is really good with interviewing and observation. Naturalistic inquiry takes skill. Figure out how to do qualitative analysis before you gather data. It is harder to analyze qualitative data than quantitative data. No software can analyze your data. *You* have to analyze your data. Lastly, have a road map from beginning to end to guide you in completing your qualitative research endeavor (Patton 2015).

8.3 Conclusion

As qualitative research continues to be conducted by experts and novices alike, more dialogue is needed to enhance the quality of the work being produced. This chapter discussed the challenges and dilemmas that new researchers encounter in different stages of a naturalistic inquiry, and made suggestions for better addressing the identified issues. It presented recommendations and approaches toward selecting a topic, exploring the literature, selecting the setting, considering ethical perspectives, choosing a methodology and research design, and collecting, managing, and analyzing data based on existing literature from experts in the field. Hopefully, it provided guidance and support for those planning to embark on designing a qualitative study for the first time, including those who are new inquirers of qualitative research.

References

Bradbury-Jones, C., Sambrook, S., and Irvine, F. (2011). Empowerment and being valued: a phenomenological study of nursing students' experiences of clinical practice. *Nurse Education Today* 31 (4): 368–372.

Dupin, C., Borglin, G., Debout, C., and Rothan-Tondeur, M. (2012). An ethnographic study of nurses' experience with nursing research and its integration into practice. *Journal of Advanced Nursing* 70 (9): 2128–2139.

Glaser, B.G. (1978). *Theoretical Sensitivity*. Sociology Press.

Martins, D.C. (2008). Experiences of homeless people in the health care delivery system: a descriptive phenomenological study. *Public Health Nursing* 25 (5): 420–430.

Mason, J. (1996). *Qualitative Researching*. Sage Publications.

Miles, M. and Huberman, A. (1984). *Qualitative Data Analysis*. Sage Publications.

Morse, J.M. and Field, P.A. (1995). *Qualitative Research Methods for Health Professionals*, 2nde. Sage Publications.

Neiswiadomy, R.M. and Bailey, C. (2018). *Foundations of Nursing Research*, 7e. Pearson Education.

O'Shea, M. and Kelly, B. (2007). The lived experiences of newly qualified nurses on clinical placement during the first six months following registration in the Republic of Ireland. *Journal of Clinical Nursing* 16 (8): 1534–1542.

Patton, M.Q. (2015). *Qualitative Research and Evaluation Methods*, 4e. Sage Publications.

Polit, D.F. and Beck, C.H. (2014). *Essentials of Nursing Research: Appraising Evidence for Nursing Practice*. Lippincott Williams & Wilkins.

Polit, D.F. and Beck, C.H. (2017). *Nursing Research: Generating and Assessing Evidence for Nursing Practice*, 10e. Wolters Kluwer Health.

Sandelowski, M. (1993). Theory unmasked: the uses and guises of theory in qualitative research. *Research in Nursing and Health* 16 (3): 213–218.

Sanjari, M., Bahramnezhad, F., Fomani, F.K. et al. (2014). Ethical challenges of researchers in qualitative studies: the necessity to develop a specific guideline. *Journal of Medical Ethics and History of Medicine* 7 (14): 1–6.

Silverman, D. (2005). *Doing Qualitative Research*, 2e. Sage Publications.

Troy, P.H., Wyness, L.A., and McAuliffe, E. (2007). Nurses' experiences of recruitment and migration from developing countries: a phenomenological approach. *Human Resources for Health* 5 (1): 15.

9

Effective Mentoring Relationships and Teamwork in Qualitative Research

Nursing is at a critical juncture in the history of the healthcare professions (Maritz and Roets 2013). The significant role of public recognition of nursing in shaping the future of healthcare demands more doctoral-prepared nurses, and thus innovative ways of educating and supporting novice nurse researchers. There is a need to prepare the future generation of researchers who will develop and advance knowledge through nursing research in order to build the scientific foundation for clinical practice, prevent disease and disability, manage and eliminate symptoms caused by illness, and enhance end-of-life and palliative care (National Institute of Nursing Research 2018). According to the Committee for Monitoring the Nation's Changing Needs for Biomedical, Behavioral, and Clinical Personnel, Board on Higher Education and Workforce, National Research Council (2005), there is evidence to suggest that a successful career in science is the result of a number of key factors across the lifespan, including knowledge, skill, and leadership development; opportunities for coaching, role modeling, and mentoring; a scientific community with peer engagement, assessment, support, and critique; and adequate support for research in all of its phases (National Research Council 2005).

Conducting a qualitative research study is a labor-intensive and complex endeavor. A dissertation or research chair or adviser is usually assigned to a doctoral student, and a mentor to novices and early-career researchers, to guide them in every step of the investigative process. Supervision has been recognized as a professional skill that requires training and monitoring (Silverman 2005). A set of clear expectations about the support and advice that an adviser can offer, and what to do when these are not met, is usually provided from early on. There are also standards of practice and structures set by institutions that must be followed in order to provide good practice.

Mentors generally have a more personal relationship with their protégés than do supervisors and advisers, who usually focus more on the academic progress of the student and serve as information resources (Eller et al. 2014; Richards and Richards 1994). One of the major differences between supervision/advising and mentoring is that the former is often task-oriented, whereas the latter is more about caring for an individual's long-term development (Eller et al. 2014). As such, a mentor's work goes beyond academic matters, combining guidance with emotional support, career advice, and role modeling to help students through graduate school and sometimes their postdoctoral training. A mentor makes an individualized, personalized effort to assist the mentee in

Fundamentals of Qualitative Phenomenological Nursing Research, First Edition. Brigitte S. Cypress.
© 2022 John Wiley & Sons Ltd. Published 2022 by John Wiley & Sons Ltd.

achieving their goals and becoming successful (Eller et al. 2014; Straus et al. 2013). It is the individualization of the efforts that makes mentoring really work. Mentors are those who are willing and able to share their experiences and expertise. They reflect on their successes and failures, and can explain what they have learned (Bird 2001). Mentorship is a close relationship that has enhanced career benefits for students, novices, and early-career qualitative researchers. Such relationships at times develop into lifelong friendships, with mentors having an emotional investment and personal interest in the success of their mentees (Richards and Richards 1994).

9.1 Mentoring Conceptual Framework

There is a dearth of literature on guidance and best practices in mentoring, and of conceptual frameworks that can guide research in this topic (Yob and Crawford 2012). Hale and Phillips (2019) assert that, to date, no theories addressing the processes involved in nurse-to-nurse mentoring have been identified. They add that research on mentoring has resulted in fragmentation of knowledge rather than conceptualization and theoretical discovery. A review of literature conducted by Yob and Crawford (2012) describes a conceptual framework that fits in mentoring of doctoral students. Two broad domains of mentoring behaviors and characteristics are identified: academic and psychosocial. The authors emphasize that for mentors, psychosocial attributes are equally as important as academic qualities. These two domains are interwoven.

The academic domain encompasses technical and informational functions of the mentor that support mentee development. The four primary attributes identified are: competence, availability, induction, and challenge. Competence includes the mentor's general knowledge in the field of expertise and their research methods. The mentor has a good grasp about specific program requirements and knows how to navigate systems and gain access to resources like experts, groups, websites, and materials. Availability includes having adequate office hours, being willing to offer extra help outside of class time, taking time to advise, spending time in conversation, and having the flexibility to meet in a variety of places. Induction involves connecting mentees to the right people, giving them access to networks and communities, and informing them on the culture of the institution and its specific processes and expectations. Challenge involves maximizing mentees' professional and personal potential, inculcating professional values and ethics, nurturing a growing sense of independence that will foster personal and professional autonomy, and teaching effective behavior and interpersonal skills. The mentor challenges the mentee to continue to grow in a friendly and collegial manner. Constructive criticisms and prompt feedback are given in a gentle manner. There also has to be a balance of advocacy and empathy, with assessment and evaluation of the novice's work, as well as early detection of flaws (Yob and Crawford 2012).

The psychosocial domain is equally important. It encompasses the skills and qualities required to establish the interpersonal relationships necessary in mentoring. The primary attributes identified are: personal qualities, communication, and emotional support. Personal qualities include trust combined with respect, openness, a genuine interest in exploring and developing the mentee's capacities, friendliness, a good sense of humor, and patience. Communication includes active listening, valuing silence, use of affirming body language, speaking the truth, mutuality, and respectful disagreement. Competence in communication is perceived by mentees as an important factor in a good mentor–mentee relationship. Aggressive and conflictual communication styles result in distrust, confusion, and poor outcomes, including a negative impact on the mentor's credibility and effectiveness. Emotional support is described as genuine caring, encouragement, accentuation of the mentee's promise and talent, affirmation and confirmation of potentials, and being a counselor and mutual confidante (Yob and Crawford 2012).

9.2 Defining the Qualities of an Ideal Mentor and Mentee

Mentoring is a professional relationship governed by the attributes, style, and chemistry of the individuals involved. Outstanding mentors: (i) exhibit admirable personal qualities, including enthusiasm, compassion, and selflessness; (ii) act as career guides, offering a vision but purposefully tailoring support to the individual mentee; (iii) make strong time commitments with regular, frequent, and high-quality meetings (accessibility); (iv) support personal/professional balance; and (v) leave a legacy regarding how to be a good mentor through role modeling and institution of policies that set global expectations and standards for mentorship (Cho et al. 2011). Altruism, honesty, trustworthiness, and active listening are good qualities identified (Straus et al. 2013). Good mentors are sincere in their dealings with mentees, understand mentees' needs, and have a well-established position within the academic community (Sambunjak et al. 2009). Mentors respond to questions and are able to articulate their requirements and expectations to mentees. Mentors expect mentees to pay attention and provide feedback regarding the adequacy of the advice they are receiving. By the same token, mentees are open to feedback, are active listeners, and are respectful of their mentor's input and time (Straus et al. 2013). According to Bird (2001), advice should be taken as a suggestion regarding a problem or set of circumstances based on a unique perspective framed by the experiences, values, and goals of the mentor. Bird (2001) states: "As a result, mentors, and mentees should expect that advisees will not necessarily follow the advice they are given. It is essential that students evaluate the advice they receive in the context of their own values, goals, needs, resources, and experience" (p. 466).

Ethical behavior is also an expectation on the part of both mentor and mentee. Mentors and mentees engage in and model ethical behavior, while openly discussing issues dealing with gray areas. Both take responsibility for their own behavior, seek out formal and informal ways of understanding the accepted norms of practice in their field, learn about ethical issues associated with the work (including the university's policies for dealing with unethical behavior), and proactively address them (Lee et al. 2015).

9.3 What to Expect of a Mentoring Relationship?

Establishing strong mentor connections is essential to success and satisfaction in any endeavor, not only in nursing but in every field, whether medicine, banking, or the arts. Humans require a relationship of caring, support, and encouragement. Mentoring entails collaboration rather than competition. It means deliberately establishing webs of relationships and caring that will connect, guide, protect, and instruct the mentee. It fosters an environment where respect, learning, support, and sharing are expectations. This is the idea behind the learning–mentoring organization described by organizational theorists (Vance 2003).

Research mentoring relationships vary considerably in their effectiveness, which is often attributed to the ability of the research mentor to shape and guide the research experience for mentees (Lee et al. 2015). Conducting a research study is not a "walk in the park," especially where it involves starting and completing a qualitative inquiry. Early-career researchers face major challenges and are usually overwhelmed by the intricacies of the research methods employed in undertaking a scholarly investigation that is appropriate and will be accepted by the scholarly community (Ellis and Levy 2009). Ellis and Levy (2009) state: "As both a consumer and producer of research, it is essential to have a firm grasp on just what is entailed in producing legitimate, valid results and conclusions" (p. 323). Not all advisers are mentors – but, in general, supervision, along with mentoring, is necessary in order for novices to be successful in their research endeavor.

Students, early-career researchers, and supervisors must first consider what to expect of one another from the early to the later stages of a qualitative research endeavor. Some of the novice's expectations are that they will be supervised, have their work read in advance, and have access to supervisors when needed, and that supervisors will be open, supportive, friendly, constructively critical, have a good knowledge of the research area, and be interested in the topic (Silverman 2005). Similarly, supervisors' expectations will include that the supervisee will work independently, be available for regular meetings, be honest about their progress, follow advice, be enthusiastic about their work, in some way be "fun" to be with, and provide surprises (Silverman 2005). The support that a supervisor gives is facilitated by an institutional structure within the department that encourages good practice. While supervision is task-oriented, mentoring adds a more personal touch to the mentee's journey, but it is both a formal and a professional relationship.

A consensus statement by the National Academy of Sciences, National Academy of Engineering & Institute of Medicine (1997) defines mentoring as a complex personal and professional relationship based on mutual interests. Such a relationship needs to be built on candor, trust, and open communication (Bird 2001; Eller et al. 2014). As in any successful, dynamic, and reciprocal relationship, compatibility, "being on the same wavelength," and "having the right chemistry" are also essential to good mentoring. According to Jackson et al. (2003), effective mentoring necessitates a certain chemistry for an appropriate interpersonal match. As a result, finding a successful mentoring relationship requires the mentee and the mentor to know about their respective working, communication, and relational styles (Jackson et al. 2003). Mentees take an active role in the formation and development of the mentoring relationship (Cho et al. 2011). They may also need to experiment with many different potential mentors to find the right match. Successful mentoring relationships are characterized by: (i) reciprocity: bi-directional mentoring, including consideration of strategies to make the relationship sustainable and mutually rewarding; (ii) mutual respect: respect for the mentor's and the mentee's time, effort, and qualifications; (iii) clear expectations: expectations should be outlined at the onset, and revisited over time; (iv) accountability: both mentor and mentee should be held accountable to these expectations; (v) personal connection: connection between the mentor and the mentee; and (vi) shared values: around the mentor's and the mentee's approach to research, clinical work, and personal life (Cho et al. 2011). Other components of an effective mentoring relationship are passion and inspiration, caring personal relationship, trust, exchange of knowledge, independence, collaboration, and role-modeling (Eller et al. 2014).

9.4 What Is a Successful Mentoring Relationship?

An effective, successful, and fruitful mentor–mentee relationship is always the goal, described as: (i) communication: including open, tactful communication and the ability to listen; (ii) commitment: to the relationship or interest over time; (iii) acceptance: of personality differences between mentor and mentee; and (iv) respect: dealing with perceived (or real) competition positively, recognizing overlapping interests, and having clarity around intellectual property (Straus et al. 2013). These factors can be classified as personal and relational factors to successful mentoring (Cho et al. 2011). There are also several contextual determinants that seem to have some influence upon the mentoring experience of mentors: cultural and mental differences, career stage, and organizational/institutional factors (Cho et al. 2011; Iancu-Haddad and Oplatka 2009).

One of the most important contextual determinants of the mentoring experience is the organizational or institutional context, although this also holds outside of this domain. Mentoring is an integral part of the mentor's responsibilities as a teacher. It is likely that teachers whose peers have responded favorably to mentoring will be encouraged to mentor, whereas those who have found themselves isolated as mentors will feel less comfortable with mentoring. The mentor's career stage and the perceived benefits of mentoring also affect the mentor–mentee relationship. Although mentors share many perceptions regardless of their career stage, Iancu-Haddad and Oplatka (2009) found some different motivations and benefits that seem to be particular to a certain stage. "Establishment career" mentors see mentoring as a kind of informal promotion, a sign that they are trusted and being given more responsibility. Iancu-Haddad and Oplatka (2009) state:

> Mid-career mentors felt that being asked to mentor was in itself a badge of
> honor, recognition of their teaching skill . . . Teachers in the late-career stage
> felt that even though they would soon retire they were passing on a legacy by
> mentoring a novice teacher . . . While teachers in the establishment career
> stage could identify with novices, older teachers mentioned the impact of the
> age gap upon their feelings. They expressed the difficulties caused by changes
> in work ethics over time and demonstrated the frustration of senior teachers
> who cannot [adjust] to the novices' way of thinking. (pp. 58–59)

Iancu-Haddad and Oplatka (2009) also explore the factors that can deter senior teachers from accepting the mentoring role. One of the predominant reasons given for refusing mentoring is time limitations. Another negative motive is related to novice teachers' conduct. Some mentors expect a novice to demonstrate dedication and cooperation.

Jackson et al. (2003) discuss troublesome mentoring relationships. Occasionally, mentors will take advantage of mentees. This violation might include taking credit for the mentee's work, or sexually harassing the mentee.

9.5 Exemplar: The Research Mentoring Process

Novice and early-career researchers, including doctoral students in general, face significant complexity in deciding on the research methods appropriate for a scholarly inquiry. They mistakenly think that the research process starts with deciding upon what type of study to pursue. On the contrary, the type of study one embarks on is based upon three related issues: the problem or phenomenon driving the investigation, the body of knowledge, and the nature of the data available (Ellis and Levy 2009). In a qualitative research endeavor, one starts with the identification of a literature-supported significant phenomenon. According to Ellis and Levy (2009), the best design cannot provide meaning to research and answer the question "Why was the study conducted?" without the anchor of a clearly identified research problem (p. 324). A mentor can assist a mentee in creating a plan if they have knowledge of the mentee's potential, allowing for a clear vision and unique perspective on the phenomenon at hand. A high standard should be set for the mentee to abide by, which will help in creating and implementing the plan (Yob and Crawford 2012).

Once a clear phenomenon has been determined, the literature should be searched for guidance on the specific methods to be followed in carrying out a study of a given type, including establishing its significance. The neophyte researcher then decides whether access to data is feasible and how to actually collect them, taking into account the ethical considerations. Access to data dictates what methods can be used. Without access to data, it is impossible for a researcher to reach any meaningful conclusions on the phenomenon of interest (Ellis and Levy 2009). The mentor should suggest the use of appropriate resources, such as a librarian, information technologist, or other experts in the field within the institution, including public organizations, existing documents, records, and archives, if necessary. An expert can also provide a wide breadth of opportunities to the mentee by introducing them to key persons, contacts, collaborators, committees, and related groups.

9.5.1 What Type of Qualitative Research Design to Choose?

Deciding on the qualitative research design to use will depend on the nature of the phenomenon being addressed. Some problems, for example, are relatively new, and require exploratory types of research, while more mature ones might better be addressed by descriptive approaches. The aim of research is to test, to revise, or to build a theory. Qualitative investigations are usually geared toward building a theory where no solid one currently exists to explain a phenomenon. The beginner investigator may opt for a grounded theory, an ethnography, a phenomenology, or a historical or case study. An expert mentor can guide the novice in what type of design and corresponding methods are appropriate for the phenomenon at hand. Another important aspect to consider is what type of data are available and accessible. Qualitative data are complex and multidimensional, and are derived from a natural setting (Ellis and Levy 2009). Data collection methods and analyses vary according to the specific research design chosen. The mentor assists by helping the mentee find their own way, leading rather than directing and drawing out the best in them (Yob and Crawford 2012).

9.5.2 What are the Questions to Ask?

There are a number of important factors that must be followed in an effective description of research methods, regardless of the type of study being conducted (Ellis and Levy 2009). In order to determine how the study will be carried out, it is necessary to answer the "what, who, how, when, where, and why" questions (Cypress 2015). These are: (i) What is going to be done? (phenomenon and research question); (ii) Who is going to do each thing to be done? (one researcher or a team); (iii) How will each thing to be done be accomplished? (research design and methods); (iv) When, and in what order, will the things to be accomplished actually be done? (time element); (v) Where will these things be done? (setting); and (vi) Why? – supported by the literature – for the answers to the what, who, how, when, and where questions (significance and review of literature) (National Academy of Sciences, National Academy of Engineering & Institute of Medicine 1997). The mentor is a significant person and expert that the novice can look up to in order to carry out the whole research process. There are a number of concrete activities that the mentor can guide the mentee in, from grant writing, selecting and gaining entry to the research site, ethical considerations, data collection and analysis, and establishing rigor to thinking critically what the study results mean, including reading and giving feedback, starting the "write-up," and revising the manuscript as needed. The mentee will also benefit from the mentor's guidance on writing for publication and preparing presentations in order to disseminate their findings.

9.6 Outcomes of the Mentoring Process

Mentoring has positive and negative outcomes on both the mentor and the mentee. Kammeyer-Mueller and Judge (2008) conducted a quantitative research synthesis focused on estimating multivariate analytical paths between mentoring and several career outcomes. They found that mentoring does have substantial effects on the job and career satisfaction of the mentor, yet factors such as core self-evaluations, tenure, and education have stronger ones. Iancu-Haddad and Oplatka (2009) articulate that mentoring may benefit the mentor in several ways: providing an opportunity for personal and professional development, enabling those in mid-career to enhance their self-esteem, and providing opportunities to pass on personal values and experiences to the next generation. They further discuss how senior professionals may view the request to mentor as validation of their status as an expert with knowledge and wisdom to share, while experienced workers approaching retirement may see mentoring as an opportunity to influence the future of their organization and make a meaningful contribution to their field. Mentoring can provide a learning experience for the mentor through self-reflection and mutual cooperation.

Mentoring may also bring about negative consequences for the mentor: a drain on their physical and mental resources, a further burden on an already busy teaching schedule, feelings of displacement, and loss of privacy. Other negative aspects of mentoring are emotional in nature, described as feelings of frustration, annoyance, anxiety, and disappointment, and concerns regarding lack of time and the pressure to carry out the mentoring role conscientiously while still being an effective teacher (Iancu-Haddad and Oplatka 2009).

For the mentee, successful mentoring results in the completion of a difficult endeavor like a dissertation, as well as future other research projects. Effective mentoring relationships at times develop into lifelong friendships and professional kinships. On the other hand, ineffective mentoring can lead to a failed completion of a research endeavor and a stained bond between expert and protégé.

9.7 Implications for Research and Formal Mentoring Programs

This chapter reveals that mentoring is both a challenge and a learning experience for both the mentor and the mentee. Mentoring involves relational interactions that are relevant and exist beyond the expectation of fulfilling a task, and the development of a mentor–mentee relationship. The mentoring relationship aims to foster the mentee's personal and professional learning and growth, to generate synergy, to inspire, and to empower, with a view to fostering increased individual performance, innovation, productivity, and achievement. According to Maritz et al. (2013), mentoring provides opportunities for the personal and professional growth of students or novices through acquisition of new skills, generation of opportunities for intellectual discourse, risk-taking, and challenges, and integration in the formal and informal research communities of practice. Based on these findings, a few recommendations can be set forth.

There is a need to assess and understand faculty members' and doctoral students' perceptions of the qualities necessary for effective mentoring, while considering the gender, cultural, and ethnic backgrounds of both parties (Yob and Crawford 2012). Academic institutions, researchers, administrators, and policy-makers need to revisit their objectives and be more aware of the benefits of mentoring for mentors, mentees, organizations, academia, and society at alarge (Iancu-Haddad and Oplatka 2009). It is evident in the literature that the institutional environment influences and plays an important role in creating a successful and productive working relationship by helping improve mentoring conditions and situations (Iancu-Haddad and Oplatka 2009). Mentors should be supported during the process through assistance and interventions that will aid in alleviating their stress, such as allowing them schedule flexibility, understanding their experiences and their emotional and coping issues, and providing them with necessary resources (Iancu-Haddad and Oplatka 2009). It will be beneficial to assign professors to students early on who will be excellent mentors (not just supervisors) that can objectively and devotedly guide their mentees into a "less painful" journey to completing a qualitative research inquiry. Mentorship programs provide students and neophytes with a supportive space in which their learning can be enhanced. They also allow for a formative social context through which to negotiate the tensions of mentoring relationships, while improving accountability and building a shared repertoire of research practice. Future research is needed to further understand and re-emphasize the attributes, ideal characteristics, and relevance of a mentor, a mentee, and the mentoring relationship as a whole, thereby confirming or disconfirming the conceptual framework (Yob and Crawford 2012).

9.8 Conclusion

This chapter presented the role of mentoring in successfully completing a scholarly inquiry that will help in equipping novices with the knowledge, skills, and confidence to navigate the difficult and long journey of undertaking a qualitative study. Different strategies for effective mentorship for both the mentor and the mentee were discussed.

References

Bird, S.J. (2001). Mentors, advisors and supervisors: Their role in teaching responsible research conduct. *Science and Engineering Ethics* 7: 455–468.

Cho, C.S., Radhika, A., Ramanan, R.A., and Feldman, M.D. (2011). Defining the ideal qualities of mentorship: a qualitative analysis of the characteristics of outstanding mentors. *American Journal of Medicine* 124: 453–458.

Cypress, B. (2015). Qualitative research: the "what,", "why," "who," and "how". *Dimensions of Critical Care Nursing* 34 (6): 356–361.

Eller, L.S., Lev, L., and Feurer, E. (2014). Key components of an effective mentoring relationship: a qualitative study. *Nurse Education Today* 34 (5): 815–820.

Ellis, T.J. and Levy, Y. (2009). Towards a guide for novice researchers on research methodology: review and proposed methods. *Issues in Informing Science and Information Technology* 6: 323–336.

Hale, R.L. and Phillips, C.A. (2019). Mentoring up: a grounded theory of nurse-to-nurse mentoring. *Journal of Clinical Nursing* 28 (1–2): 159–172.

Iancu-Haddad, D. and Oplatka, I. (2009). Mentoring novice teachers: motives, process, and outcomes from the mentor's point of view. *New Educator* 5 (45): 45–65.

Jackson, V.A., Palepu, A., Szalacha, L. et al. (2003). Having the right chemistry: a qualitative study of mentoring in academic medicine. *Academic Medicine* 7 (8): 328–334.

Kammeyer-Mueller, J.D. and Judge, T.A. (2008). A quantitative review of mentoring research: test of a model. *Journal of Vocational Behavior* 72 (3): 269–283.

Lee, S.P., McGee, R., Pfund, C., and Branchaw, J. (2015). Mentoring up: learning to manage your mentoring relationships. In: *The Mentoring Continuum* (ed. G. Wright). The Graduate School Press of Syracuse University.

Maritz, J., Visagie, R., and Johnson, B. (2013). External group coaching and mentoring: building a research community of practice at a university of technology. *Perspectives in Education* 31 (4): 155–167.

Maritz, J.E. and Roets, L. (2013). A virtual appreciative coaching and mentoring programme to support novice nurse researchers in Africa. *Journal of Physical, Health Education, Recreation and Dance (AJPHERD)* September (Supplement 1): 80–92.

National Research Council (2005). *Advancing the Nation's Health Needs: NIH Research Training Programs*. The National Academies Press.

National Academy of Sciences, National Academy of Engineering & Institute of Medicine. (1997). Adviser, teacher, role model, friend: on being a mentor to students in science and engineering. Available from https://www.nap.edu/readingroom/books/mentor (accessed May 10, 2021).

National Institute of Nursing Research. (2018). Nursing research develops knowledge. Available from https://www.ninr.nih.gov/ (accessed May 10, 2021).

Richards, T.J. and Richards, L. (1994). Using computers in qualitative research. In: *Handbook of Qualitative Research* (eds. N.K. Denzin and Y.S. Lincoln), 273–285. Sage Publications.

Sambunjak, D., Straus, S.E., and Marusic, A. (2009). A systematic review of qualitative research on the meaning and characteristics of mentoring in academic medicine. *Journal of General Internal Medicine* 25 (1): 72–78.

Silverman, D. (2005). *Doing Qualitative Research*, 2nde. Sage Publications.

Straus, S.E., Johnson, M.O., Marquez, C., and Feldman, M.D. (2013). Characteristics of successful and failed mentoring relationships: a qualitative study across two academic health centers. *Academic Medicine* 88 (1): 82–89.

Vance, C.C. (2003). Mentoring at the age of chaos. *Nurse Leader 8* (3): 7–14.

Yob, I.M. and Crawford, L.C. (2012). Conceptual framework for mentoring doctoral students. *Higher Learning Research in Communication* 2 (2): 34–47.

VI Phenomen-ological Outcomes and Applications in Evidence-Based Practice, Policy, and Theory

10

Outcomes of Qualitative Phenomenological Research
Linking Findings to Evidence-Based Practice, Policy, and Theory

10.1 Asking "Meaning Questions" in Evidence-Based Reviews and the Utility of Qualitative Research Findings in Practice

"Meaning questions" in EBP systematic reviews have been presented by experts for some time – but their use is remarkably scant in the literature. Findings from reviews utilizing qualitative research questions might allow researchers to expand the array of variables that contribute to the production of specific outcomes across multiple settings. The empirical results from randomized controlled trials (**RCTs**) are always considered the "gold standard" – but these should be supplemented with other methods, including in-depth qualitative approaches that can illuminate important nuances of practice (Kozleski 2017).

Qualitative research is *empirical,* stemming from experience and/or observation. It produces knowledge about perspectives, settings, and techniques, and involves the systematic use of specific research skills and tools (Brantlinger et al. 2005). Naturalistic investigations also represent a legitimate mode of social and human science exploration, about which perhaps little is known (Cypress 2015). To call qualitative methods "empirical" still produces much debate among researchers even today. Qualitative methods allow for new discoveries in the moment, unlike more restrictive quantitative data sources such as surveys that are structured for participants to respond *to* rather than *with* the research team. Kozleski (2017) states: "Importantly, qualitative methods situate research participants in the role of 'story-teller,' providing participants the opportunity to highlight issues that are important but may not have occurred to researchers" (p. 24). Qualitative research provides essential information about the implementation

Fundamentals of Qualitative Phenomenological Nursing Research, First Edition. Brigitte S. Cypress.
© 2022 John Wiley & Sons Ltd. Published 2022 by John Wiley & Sons Ltd.

of EBP, including its critical components, the ways that it affects participants, and key players' perceptions. The sheer proliferation of these types of health research has made qualitative findings difficult to dismiss and has generated urgent calls to incorporate them into the evidence-based scientist's practice process (Cypress 2012).

Qualitative methods apply to EBP approaches such as systematic reviews that start with a "meaning" problem/population–intervention–comparison intervention–outcomes (PICO) question. As far back as 2009, Odom asserted that there have to be new innovations or changes in the way we implement EBP research steps and practices. He emphasized that the usual EBP practices are no longer contemporary, "hot," or *wired*, or are not visionary (*tired*), and representations are passé or no longer at the forefront of the most active thinking about issues (*expired*) (Odom 2009). Wired topics are "hot" topics (Odom 2009), are at the forefront of the field, represent the next steps in the field, and thus move the field forward. Topics for EBP reviews have included etiology, diagnosis, therapy, prevention, and prognosis for many years. It is time for reviews that use "meaning questions." Old approaches are still relevant or essential, but are no longer sufficient to foster a move from science to application or practice (Odom 2009). Kozleski (2017) summarizes this and states: "When EBPs remains a description of idealized practice rather than actively engaged practices that produce more knowledge about the conditions for improvement and successful outcomes, the research community remains aloof from the complex work of improvement and innovation and damages the odds of the diffusion of EBPs" (p. 21). New approaches have evolved, allowing investigators to assess the contributions of qualitative studies to the landscape of scientific thought and practice (Kozleski 2017).

10.1.1 Relevance of Qualitative Evidence-Based Systematic Reviews

Systematic reviews are one of the cornerstones of EBP. They are helpful for clinicians who want to integrate research findings into their daily practices, for patients who want to make well-informed choices about their own care, and for professional medical societies and other organizations that want to develop clinical practice guidelines (Institute of Medicine 2011). The results of systematic reviews can demonstrate where knowledge is lacking, and thus guide future research (Gopalakrishnan and Ganeshkumar 2013). However, some proponents of quantitative research and scientists still subscribe to the idea that the only true approach to scientific inquiry is through conducting RCTs. Advocates of qualitative research are often troubled by the use of hierarchies of evidence that assume RCTs to be the most reliable form, which thereby devalue or exclude qualitative studies from many systematic reviews or from any regard at all, let alone consideration as best evidence (Cypress 2012; Noyes 2010; Pearson 2010). Naturalistic research is perceived as unscientific and anecdotal by many investigators. Personal experience and its narratives are often characterized as ungeneralizable and a poor basis for making scientific decisions. Qualitative studies are also ranked lower and weaker, along with descriptive, evaluative, and case studies, compared with other research designs that examine and administer interventions. Almost invariably, they are regarded as the lowest level of research, being of a provisional nature to be used first pending better, "real" ways of producing evidence. However, not all phenomena are amenable to quantitative experimentation and measurement. Clinical experience, based on personal observation, reflection, and judgment, is also needed to translate scientific results into treatment of individual patients. "Good evidence" goes further than the results of RCTs. Qualitative research methods that involve understanding of human or social problems are developed to fill the gap, including the use of "meaning questions" in systematic evidence-based reviews.

Evidence-based systematic reviews usually utilize PICO questions in the areas of etiology, diagnosis, therapy, prevention, and prognosis. The use of "meaning questions" is sparse. Analyzing and synthesizing evidence using "meaning questions" is important in that it incorporates patients' voices and experiences into the process of EBP (Cypress 2012). "Meaning questions" are part of clinical inquiry and are appropriate for use (Cypress 2011). These types of questions are qualitative in nature and are asked in order to determine meaning, to provide insight and scope to a phenomenon, and to appreciate a specific population's experience (Brantlinger et al. 2005). A qualitative PICO question focuses on in-depth perspectives and experiences. Its use can explore, illuminate, and enrich the understanding of a particular EBP question or of a phenomenon that needs to be described in a contextual, holistic way that cannot be provided through quantification or measurability. Such deeper understanding of a phenomenon can be attained only through an inquiry using a qualitative perspective.

Several alternative search strategy tools to PICO have been proposed for use with qualitative research. First are **SPICE** (Setting, Population, Intervention, Comparison, and Evaluation), promoted by the Joanna Briggs Institute for qualitative systematic reviews, and **ECLIPSE** (Expectation, Client group, Location, Impact, Professionals, ServicE). Neither meets the full requirements of the qualitative research paradigm, nor are they suitable for use with more general qualitative research questions (Cooke et al. 2012). Next, **CIMO** (Context–Intervention– Mechanism–Outcome), developed for management questions, might hold potential within realist synthesis (Cooke et al. 2012). Finally, **SPIDER** (Sample, Phenomenon of Interest, Design, Evaluation, Research type) was designed to overcome the difficulties of using PICO when searching for qualitative and mixed-methods research for metasynthesis by including the "research type (R)" category (Cooke et al. 2012).

The PICO tool has spread from its early origins in epidemiology to become a fundamental tool in both EBP and systematic reviews (Cooke et al. 2012), but there is still a lack of synthesis of evidence using "meaning questions" in the literature.

This chapter focuses on EBP reviews used to synthesize qualitative research findings using "meaning questions" as a PICO format. Two exemplars of evidence-based reviews utilizing qualitative PICO questions follow.

10.1.2 Exemplars: Two Evidenced-Based Systematic Reviews Using "Meaning Questions"

I conducted two evidence-based systematic reviews using "meaning questions" (Cypress 2011, 2013), following the Scottish Intercollegiate Guidelines Network (SIGN, 2008) and evidence-based concepts from Melnyk and Fineout-Overholt (2019) for categorization of levels of evidence in both cases. My topics were transfer or discharge of the critically ill patient to the regular medical-surgical floor and family conference and/or meeting in the intensive care unit (**ICU**).

10.1.2.1 Family Conference in the ICU

Family conference and/or meeting is one of the recommendations presented by the American College of Critical Care Medicine (ACCM, 2017) under the shared decision-making model. The guidelines set forth by the ACCM emphasize that routine interdisciplinary family conferences should be used in the ICU to improve family satisfaction with communication and trust in clinicians and to reduce conflict between clinicians and family members (Davidson et al. 2017). Family conference and/or meeting is not diligently done in actual practice, nor is it an automatic standard protocol in ICUs. Rather, it is carried out in silos or on a "needs basis," if a patient is doing "poorly," at the end of life, or unable to make decisions on their own related to their medical condition or when a family is labeled as "problematic or demanding." Family conferences also take place when the ICU team believes that it is time to consider withdrawing life support (Hurd and Curtis 2015). Hurd and Curtis (2015) state: "In this context, we run the risk of inadvertently encouraging a hidden curriculum that implies that when family conferences are done well, patients and families elect to withdraw life-sustaining treatments" (p. 470). Families of critically ill patients often do not understand even basic information about the patient's diagnosis, prognosis, or treatment (Kodali 2014). Physicians often miss opportunities to listen to, acknowledge, and address the emotions of families, and do not explain surrogate decision-making. Improved communication with families of patients admitted to an ICU has been shown to improve family satisfaction and psychological well-being, reduce length of stay, and, where appropriate, result in earlier withdrawal of life-sustaining interventions and increase referrals to hospice (Kodali 2014). Family conferences should be conducted at regular intervals to help the critical care team understand the patient's and family's perspectives, learn their values and preferences, and thus tailor the plan of care to their specific circumstances. This is a key step toward aligning with patients and families, and allows the team to "walk on the same path" as them and meet their needs (Hurd and Curtis 2015).

I reviewed research studies related to family conference and/or meeting during critical illness in the ICU (Cypress 2011). The PICO questions that guided this study were: "How do the family members of the adult and pediatric critically ill patients (P) perceive (O) family conferences and/or meetings (I) during ICU admission (T)?" and, "How do the health care staff of the adult and pediatric critical inpatients (P) perceive (O) family conferences and/or meetings (I) during ICU admission (T)?" These questions are qualitative in nature, and cannot be answered using the quantitative PICO templates (etiology, diagnosis, therapy, prevention, and prognosis). "Meaning questions" do not require a comparison intervention in their statement. Rather, explicating family members' and healthcare staff's perceptions of their experiences of family conference and/or meeting is necessary. Synthesis of evidence showed that the family members and healthcare staff perceived that family conference and/or meeting had a positive impact on the communication taking place during conferences, increasing

Table 10.1 Family conference and/or meeting in the ICU: family and healthcare outcomes.

Category	Outcome
Communication	Understanding of medical condition and status
	Understanding of goals of care
	Understanding of prognosis
	Understanding of what to expect during the dying process
	Understanding of quality of life
	Clinician accessibility to patients and families
	Consistency between decisions and care
	Educational enhancement and greater awareness of issues important to end-of-life care on the staff
Decision-making	Awareness of options and choices, burdens and benefits
	Earlier consensus around goals of care for dying patients
	Transition from curative to palliative
	Assurance of patient comfort/pain management
	Withdrawal of life support (results in decreased length of stay in ICU)
	Death and dying
Family support	Valuing of family's input
	Easing of emotional burdens/emotional support and active listening
	Spiritual support
	Respect for beliefs, preferences, and family readiness
	Presence at bedside
	Support for decision-making
Family satisfaction	Communication and accessibility of information
	Assurance of non-abandonment before death
	Alleviation of patient's suffering
	Support for family's decisions about end-of-life care
	Support for family's decision to withdraw or not withdraw life support
	Family ratings of conflict with physician

Source: Adapted from Cypress, B. (2011). Family conference in the intensive care unit. *Dimension of Critical Care Nursing*, 30(5): 246–255.

family support, decision-making, and satisfaction. A summary of these findings is presented in Table 10.1. My results also showed that there is a lack of high-quality, well-conducted RCTs on family conference in the ICU. A review of the literature revealed that most existing studies are conducted in pediatric critical care rather than in adult ICUs.

10.1.2.2 The Critically Ill Patient and Transfer to the Medical-Surgical Floor

Patient discharge from the ICU and transfer to the regular medical-surgical floor is a positive step in terms of their physical and physiological recovery. However, research shows that there are varied negative consequences as well. Transition from the ICU to a general ward is a stress- and anxiety-producing event for patients and their families (Cypress 2013; Jodaki et al. 2017). Discharge is equally as traumatic as admission (Cypress 2013). There are also a myriad of physical, psychological/emotional, and environmental sequelae, as well as effects in the provision of care (Brown et al. 2018; Buchner et al. 2015; Cypress 2013; Kramer et al. 2013; National Transitions of Care Coalition 2020).

The discharge of patients from the ICU to a medical-surgical floor is a vulnerable and challenging transition. This is attributable to many factors including caring for patients with the highest acuity of illness in the hospital, transitioning from a resource-rich environment to one with fewer resources and a lower nurse-to-patient ratio (multi-professional and inter-specialty), lack of standardized discharge procedures, and high frequency of verbal and written communication failures among providers and between providers, patients, and family members (Stelfox et al. 2017). Studies still show a growing body of evidence suggesting that transition of care is associated with medical errors, adverse events, poor patient satisfaction, increased healthcare costs, and increased mortality (Brown et al. 2018; Buchner et al. 2015; Cypress 2013; Kramer et al. 2013; National Transitions of Care Coalition 2020).

I systematically reviewed the effects of ICU transfer or discharge to medical-surgical floors on adult critically ill patients, their family members, and their nurses (Cypress 2013). Two "meaning" PICO questions guided this evidence-based review: "How do the adult critically ill patients and their families perceive transfer or discharge from ICU?" and, "How do the nurses perceive transfer or discharge of adult critically ill patients from ICU?" No comparison of interventions was included, but instead I conducted an exploration of the patients', family members', and nurses' perceptions of their experiences of transfer and discharge from the ICU.

The phenomenon under review, derived from the PICO questions, was the experience of patients, their families, and nurses within the context of ICU transfer and discharge to the medical-surgical floors, which is qualitative in nature. Aligned with the qualitative essence of the topic, it is appropriate that there were more naturalistic studies included in the review, as compared with the quantitative investigations based on the set inclusion and exclusion criteria for samples. The PICO questions cannot be fully answered by research focusing on quantification and measurement of variables. An exploration, description, and understanding of the phenomenon at hand is thus fitting. The 11 qualitative evidences helped explicate the answers to the PICO questions. Discharge of patients from the ICU and transfer to the medical-surgical floor has a myriad of impacts on the patient, their family members, and their nurses. Most of the significant effects noted are negative sequelae classified as physical, psychological/emotional, environmental, and effects on provision of care. A summary of the findings is presented in Table 10.2.

Table 10.2 Outcomes of transfer and discharge from ICU for patients, family members, and nurses.

Category	Physical Responses	Psychological/Emotional Responses	Environmental Stressors	Provision of Care
Patients	Positive: will be free from sleeping difficulties Negative: weakness, pain, appetite changes, altered sleeping pattern, physical dependency, experience of dreams, worries, inability to eat, drink or care for themselves independently; feeling upset after seeing their reflection in the mirror for the first time following ICU, inability to move, change position or walk leading to anxiety that they will be bedbound thereafter	Positive: felt that the act of leaving the ICU is the most positive aspect of transfer; the transfer from ICU is a sign of progress; feeling "better," "happy," "better," and "relieved;" discharge from ICU seen as a positive step forward and indicative of recovery; the act of leaving the ICU is the most positive aspect of transfer; desire for more control over their recovery Negative: memories (real and unreal), unpleasant dreams, fear, difficulty concentrating, detachment, acceptance and mixed feeling; feeling confused or vulnerable anxious, nervous, worried, unhappy, transfer stress and anxiety for leaving a protected environment, translocation stress, traumatic experience for transfer, uncertainty, uncertain expectations of the future, concerns and worries, memory loss, lack of confidence in self and others, worries about effects on relatives, sense of sudden abandonment, pervasive feelings of vulnerability and helplessness, loss of importance and ambivalence about the experience, emotional dependency, need to feel safe and protected, felt that spouse is not truly empathetic	Positive: happy to be detached from monitors and invasive devices, noise, lights, lack of space and to be away from so many sick people, lack of privacy and visitor restrictions Negative: uncertain expectations about the ward and environment, ongoing physical effect	Positive: felt safer in ICU, liked the staff and the constant presence of nurses and rapid response to their needs Negative: concerns about nursing care and support in the floors like feeding, sudden change in communication and level of care like less observation and monitoring and less care, worries about long time to obtain assistance in the floors, concerns about rehabilitation from critical care

(Continued)

Table 10.2 (Continued)

Category	Physical Responses	Psychological/Emotional Responses	Environmental Stressors	Provision of Care
Family Members	None	Positive: feeling "better," "happy," "better," and "relieved that the family member is leaving ICU;" felt that the act of leaving the ICU is the most positive aspect of transfer; the transfer from the ICU as a sign of progress; discharge from ICU seen as a positive step forward and indicative of recovery; the act of leaving the ICU is the most positive aspect of transfer Negative: anxious, nervous, scared, worried, unhappy, stressed, sense of sudden abandonment, pervasive feelings of vulnerability and helplessness, loss of importance and ambivalence about the experience, concern about a lack of security	Positive: happy to be free from visitor restrictions, lack of privacy and lack of space	Positive: felt that their family member is safer in ICU, liked the staff in ICU and the constant presence of nurses and rapid response to their needs Negative: worried about level of care like less observation and monitoring and less care in the floors; worries about long time to obtain assistance

Category	Physical Responses	Psychological/Emotional Responses	Environmental Stressors	Provision of Care
Nurses	None	Negative: Sense of dread, depressed	Negative: Concern about equipment and resources	Positive: *"being perceptive and adjustable"*: assessing individual needs, individual care planning, educational/informational support, emotional/psychological support, assistive activities; *"preparing for a change"*: elicit trust, make the unknown known, attempt to implement the patient's own strengths; *"promoting recovery"*: creating an alliance, reinforcing the patients will, orienting and integrating Negative: concern about communication (handover), concern about the condition of patient on discharge from ICU, perceived discharge planning as time-consuming, felt uncertainty about the patient's condition, and lacked a clear idea of the responsibilities in the process

Source: Adapted from Cypress, B. (2013). Transfer out of intensive care: an evidence-based literature review. *Dimension of Critical Care Nursing*, 32(5): 244–261.

10.1.3 Other Strategies for Qualitative Research Evidence Synthesis

Beyond the PICO questions, there are other strategies toward qualitative evidence synthesis (**QES**). Thorne et al. (2004) presented and reflected on their own approaches to qualitative synthesis approaches. They realized the confusion about the representation and outcomes of these inquiries and were aware of the diverse and complex methodological techniques for synthesizing qualitative evidence and the issue of rigor, but they nonetheless aimed for a common standard in order for this endeavor to be a credible scholarly enterprise.

Noblit and Hare (1988) published a classic methodological monograph using *metaethnographic synthesis*. The strategies they used involved interpretation, proposal of a theory of explanation, and the realization that there are multiple possible forms for a metaethnographic synthesis, namely: reciprocal, refutation, and line of argument. Kearney (1998) and Thorne (2001) described their explicit methodological techniques for qualitative health research synthesis in the form of formal *grounded theory* and *metastudy* approaches. Sandelowski (2004) considered qualitative metasynthesis as one kind of systematic review and *qualitative research integration*. Qualitative metasynthesis, according to Sandelowski and Barroso (2003), is an *interpretive integration of qualitative findings* that are themselves interpretive syntheses of data, including phenomenologies, ethnographies, grounded theories, and other integrated and coherent descriptions or explanations of phenomena, events, or cases. Such interpretive syntheses of data are considered to be hallmarks of qualitative research (Thorne et al. 2004).

In summary, these researchers used metaethnography, grounded theory, metastudy, and metasynthesis with an interpretive integration perspective as techniques for QES.

10.1.4 Utilizing Qualitative Findings

Qualitative research findings are the informational content or thematic synthesis of naturalistic studies, descriptions, and explanations, or other integrated and coherent interpretations that researchers produce from the analysis of data generated in or from interviews, observations, documents, and artifacts (Sandelowski and Leeman 2012). Analysis and synthesis of the literature on a topic from systematic evidence-based reviews using "meaning questions" also yield qualitative findings. The literature on the utility of qualitative findings is evident from the late 1990s and 2000s, but rather limited thereafter.

Qualitative methods have undeniably become a standard way in which researchers generate knowledge pertinent to nursing practice (Sandelowski and Leeman 2012). The issue that always arises is that qualitative findings are perceived as preliminary to quantitative studies, cannot stand alone, are not generalizable, and can't be applied to entire populations, but rather are tailored to unique individuals in their specific contexts. Qualitative findings, however, can be complete by themselves (Miller 2010). This gap has always been apparent to researchers who anticipate that their research products will be used to facilitate informed decision-making by clinicians, resulting in improved client or population health outcomes. Naturalistic inquiries have much to contribute to the appropriateness of care. Contextual factors influence how successfully programs or policies are carried out. There is an important role for qualitative research methods derived from qualitative approaches (Jack 2006). Qualitative investigators must be assertive in affirming the value of their work by increasing awareness among clinicians and decision-makers about the different ways in which qualitative evidence can be used and applied in practice.

The state of the science has progressed to a point where qualitative research should no longer be viewed primarily as a precursor to quantitative studies. Qualitative research in the twenty-first century plays a critical role in solidifying the *evidence base* and foundation for quantitative studies (Squires and Dorsen 2018). Qualitative research can provide "knowledge for use," offering an understanding both of social processes and of how they may be modified in the pursuit of desired ends. The impact of qualitative findings, although pervasive, has the potential to influence practice. Nevertheless, the question of "application" remains. How can the findings of studies based on narratives from a few informants be applied to caring situations with other patients (Nordgren et al. 2008). The key strategy in enhancing the accessibility and usability of qualitative health research findings is first to write in the language of the readers toward whom they are directed (Sandelowski and Leeman 2012).

Sandelowski and Leeman (2012) suggest some strategies to enhance the accessibility and usability of qualitative health research findings, including translating findings into thematic sentences and applying the language of intervention and implementation. First, there is no common understanding of *theme* among qualitative researchers, and no clear line between qualitative content and thematic analysis. Knowing the difference between a theme and a topic is foundational to the crafting of accessible findings. The identification of themes is also foundational to qualitative research of all kinds. "Intervention talk," according to Sandelowski and Leeman (2012), can serve explicitly to emphasize the utility of qualitative findings; that is, to show exactly where, how, and why research and practice might be changed to improve some health outcome. For example, qualitative findings about how people experience and manage an illness can be articulated as offering a theory on the problem or a rationale to support why the patient opted to, or did not opt to, receive a particular treatment. Findings should also be presented in the results sections of research or review reports within an implementation framework or use the discussion section to illustrate how the results might contribute to the knowledge of context required effectively to implement new interventions or practices (Sandelowski and Leeman 2012). It is paramount to clearly articulate the outcomes of qualitative research to both funding agencies and decision-makers, and to develop context-specific strategies illustrating how the findings can be used by clinicians and policy-makers (Sandelowski 2004). However, effecting change in practice is a complex matter. According to Morris et al. (2011), it takes an average of 17 years for research evidence to reach clinical practice.

Effecting change in professional practice is complex and difficult to execute successfully (Roberts and Barber 2001). Conventional continuing education has shown that single strategies have little effect on translating knowledge into practice. It is evident that education must be reinforced by other strategies and that a combination of strategies is the most effective approach. Multifaceted interventions are also necessary in order to change practice, including coordinated implementation of active methods such as the combination of continuing education, clinical practice guidelines, good project management by senior staff, and individual ownership. Educational strategies can include seminars, formal presentations, workshops, and informal discussions (Roberts and Barber 2001). Findings from a study of healthcare professionals might also indicate that an implementation problem lies at the level of the *system* and not of the professionals working within that system, thereby requiring implementation processes that target *system redesign* (Sandelowski and Leeman 2012). The utility of qualitative findings can also be discussed from the perspective that research utilization may be *instrumental* (concrete applications in practice protocols), *conceptual* (cognitive applications through new insights and understandings of situations), or *symbolic* (use of findings to legitimize a policy or practice approach) (Estabrooks 1999a, b; Kearney 2001; Nordgren et al. 2008).

10.1.4.1 *Instrumental Utilization*

Instrumental utilization refers to the concrete application of findings that have been made into new forms such as clinical guidelines, standards of care, policy decisions, appraisal tools, algorithms, and intervention protocols (Miller 2010), including questionnaire development, program evaluation processes (Kearney 2001; Morse 2001), and the development of assessment guidelines from qualitatively derived theories (Kearney 2001; Morse et al. 1998; Olson 2001). Qualitative phenomenological findings, for example, have demonstrated independent instrumental utility in leading to key changes in family presence in ICUs.

The results of the two exemplar studies in the ICU (Cypress 2010, 2013) eventually led to recommendations that support recognizing the patient and family as active co-participants in the patient's medical care, encouraging family member presence, and creating institutional policies for patient- and family-centered care. These findings, and the policy created, were put into practice directly by educating nurses and physicians on the importance of family presence during critical illness, and thus encouraging them to incorporate it in their daily clinical practice with the aim of improving patient and family outcomes.

10.1.4.2 *Conceptual Utilization*

The conceptual use of research refers to a process of enlightenment whereby findings still influence decision-maker actions, but in a more indirect and less specific manner (Jack 2006). Conceptual utilization is the least tangible and most questionable example of research utilization (Sandelowski 2004). It does not entail an observable action at all, but rather a change in the way users *think* about problems, persons, or events. The action happens in the user who is newly informed, but this change may not be noticeable to anyone, nor have any evident impact. Despite conceptual utilization being intangible, it can alter how a user *thinks* about providing care (Miller 2010). It may be a precursor to instrumental utilization, as users develop the capacity to articulate the change experience and to translate it into a more observable or material form (Sandelowski 2004).

The results of the two exemplar studies in the ICU (Cypress 2010, 2013) were useful in increasing nurses' *understanding* of patients' and family members' experiences, thereby allowing for more specific tailored interventions in care in the context of family presence during critical illness with the potential to improve outcomes. For instance, involving the family in the plan of care and making them active participants, allowing them to bring pictures of the patient to the bedside, empathizing with the family, and engaging in advocacy will help bring about these goals and potentially improve the care provided to critically ill patients in intensive care.

10.1.4.3 Symbolic Utilization

Qualitative research findings may also be used symbolically by decision-makers to validate a position, program, service, or policy (Sandelowski 2004). Symbolic utilization is less visible and concrete than the other forms and does not result in a true practice change per se; rather, findings are used as a persuasive or political tool to legitimate a position or practice. Although its actionability resides largely in talk, symbolic utilization may be a precursor to instrumental utilization as a change in practice may ultimately result from this form of use (Miller 2010; Sandelowski 2004). The "stories" that emerge from qualitative research are important tools for symbolic use, and will move individuals to action (Sandelowski 2004). Symbolic utilization may be perceived negatively or seen as socially unacceptable (Jack 2006), but when research is sought to justify a decision, it may influence positive outcomes.

For example, the narratives from the patients and their families about family presence during cardio-pulmonary resuscitation, invasive procedures, family conferences, and rounds from the two exemplar phenomenological studies (Cypress 2010, 2013) were presented to the ICU staff, including nurses, physicians, the management team, and ancillary personnel. Although they received some negative opinions and resistance from members of the ICU team, they may still symbolically help change staff perceptions and move them toward implementing family presence in the ICU, eventually helping improve patient and family outcomes.

It is evident that qualitative research findings are geared most obviously to conceptual and symbolic utilization and less to instrumental utilization (Sandelowski 2004). EBP is oriented to empirical (observable action) and interventionist perspectives. Naturalistic investigations are usually perceived as less instrumentally useful. Sandelowski (2004) argues that instrumental utility is face utility. What has no face utility has no utility at all. Thus, researchers should enhance and emphasize the instrumental utility of qualitative research findings and make the value of symbolic and conceptual utilization more apparent. Qualitative research findings close the gap not only between understanding and action, but also between efficacy (or what works in research) and effectiveness (or what works in practice) (Sandelowski 2004).

10.1.5 Afterthoughts

Qualitative research and review findings are valued as part of the evidence for policy and practice. Findings from qualitative research and systematic reviews provide nurses with information allowing them to develop and improve professional care through the discovery of meanings of human experiences and contextual factors. These findings have an impact on interventions and suggest hypotheses that can be tested in future research. EBP affirms that scientific knowledge should be appraised and applied in practice. Topics of systematic reviews are predominantly about etiology, diagnosis, therapy, prevention, and prognosis of disease conditions – and very rarely about the meanings that patients, families, and healthcare providers attribute to their voices and their experiences of illness and health. Qualitative research and review findings are also perceived as less instrumentally useful. Naturalistic researchers must be assertive in affirming the value of their work by increasing awareness among clinicians and decision-makers about the different ways in which qualitative evidence can be used and applied in practice and emphasizing its instrumental utility.

10.2 Policy as an Outcome of Phenomenological Research

As early as the 1990s, there was a paradigm shift toward a more holistic, human-centered perspective and social context as shaping health, taking account of local, macro-level political and economic influences. This called for increased qualitative research, and for heightened visibility of its analysis (Muecke 1997). Barriers and social determinants of health, quality of life, diversity, the value of voice, and the political and social determinants of care, including gender, social literacy, and patients' values and preferences, caught the attention of scholars of social sciences in the search for exploration and understanding, with the aim of contributing to social change. However, qualitative research is ambiguously placed as a source of evidence for policy, and is routinely excluded from evidence review and policy development (Graham and McDermott 2016). It is often deemed less relevant than quantitative research (if not irrelevant) because it does not provide prescriptions for best practices or claim to offer "proof" that a given policy will lead to specific outcomes (Dumas and Anderson 2014). In spite of the criticisms, findings from naturalistic studies have been increasingly used to inform policy development, significantly helping affect change.

10.2.1 Enhancing Health Policy through Qualitative Research

One key dimension of equity in health is that researchers are able to disseminate their findings, which are taken into account in a fair and just manner, so that they can inform health policy and programs (Daniels et al. 2016). Qualitative research combines the power of stories with methodological rigor, providing policy-makers with important information about the complexity of problems and suggesting possible solutions (Tolman et al. 2005). Naturalistic inquiries have been challenging the notion of singular truth and objectivity and aiming toward an understanding of the structures, processes, and indicators of health and illness. Knowing these aspects through naturalistic inquiries enables the investigator to link their findings to governmental policies (Morse 1997).

Qualitative research offers a range of methods through which "real-life" experiences can be factored into policy-making. A greater appreciation of the value of qualitative approaches in the study of healthcare systems and policy can only improve decision-making in our age of high political consciousness and rapid information availability (Daniels et al. 2016). Daniels et al. (2016) state: "The methodological diversity in qualitative research not only generates new evidence and knowledge for health systems policy, planning and practice, but also incorporates approaches to engage and participate with communities (and users of services) to utilize evidence and solutions to create change" (p. 3). The reflexive process of qualitative research creates new knowledge and action, influenced by understanding of history, culture, and local context embedded in social relationships. The qualitative research community has also been working to develop ways of inserting qualitative findings into the evidence base of policy. So, what would help link health research to policy formulation? How could the demand for research among policymakers and program planners be increased (Morse 1997).

Capacity enhancement is important. There should be partnership not only with academia but also with community organizations and policy-makers in the formulation of research questions and the planning and conduct of health programs. This also requires research infrastructure, technical backup, long-term financial commitment, support for innovative thinking, collaboration, and networking (Muecke, 1997). Participatory action research (**PAR**), for example, has provided a voice in research for marginalized groups. This approach has also contributed evidence on environmental determinants of health, barriers and enablers in managing ill health, and learning about the roles and social relationships contributing to effective prevention and care (Daniels et al. 2016). Systematic reviews have been increasingly used as a tool for assessing the quality of qualitative studies (Graham and McDermott 2016) and the use of meaning questions in evidence-based reviews (Cypress 2011, 2013). Systematic reviews are held up as the gold standard for evaluating and synthesizing evidence from observational studies, both quantitative and qualitative (Graham and McDermott 2016). Examples of the impact of systematic reviews of naturalistic inquiries and qualitative research in policy-making are presented in this section.

10.2.2 Use of Participatory Action Research in the Development of a Clinical Pharmacy Support Model for Nurses and their Clients in an Australian Home Nursing Service

Elliott et al. (2017) used co-creation and PAR design to develop a collaborative, person-centered model of clinical pharmacy support for community nurses and their medication management clients in a large, non-profit home nursing service in Melbourne, Australia. This approach was chosen because it included active involvement of relevant stakeholders and consumers during its design and implementation to understand their world and insure that research outcomes were appropriate to identified needs. The aims were to improve access to clinical pharmacy services, enhance interdisciplinary teamwork, and help address problems with medication management and medication safety. Participants included focus groups containing 27 older people, 18 carers, 53 nurses, 15 general practitioners (GPs), and 7 community pharmacists. The older people belonged to the vulnerable population that needs help in managing health and illness, which can be best approached through the chosen qualitative design, thus contributing to effective prevention and care. Data collection involved feedback and reflections from minutes, notes, and transcripts from project team meetings, clinical pharmacists' reflective diaries and interviews, meetings with community nurses, reference group meetings, and interviews. The study yielded significant findings, and afforded change in pharmacy practice.

A collaborative, person-centered clinical pharmacy model that addressed the needs of clients, carers, nurses, and other stakeholders was successfully developed. This model allows nurses to refer directly to pharmacists, enabling timely resolution of medication issues. Direct care was provided to 84 older people over a 15-month implementation period. The model is likely to have applicability to home nursing services nationally and internationally (Elliott et al. 2017).

10.2.3 Female Adolescent Sexuality and the Place of Qualitative Research in Policy-Making

Tolman et al. (2005) reviewed qualitative studies on adolescent gender inequality and described key findings that can be used to inform sexuality education policies. Policy aimed at the eradication of gender inequality in U.S. public schools began with the passing of Title IX of the Education Amendments in 1972. However, up to the mid-2000s, this amendment did not address the gender inequality that has been identified in sexuality education curriculum (Tolman et al. 2005).

In 2004, a special hearing of the U.S. Senate on abstinence-only education in public school classrooms was conducted in Harrisburg, Pennsylvania. Supporters of abstinence-only education presented statistical data and stories from adolescents and authoritative advocates, including excerpts from student letters and personal observations about changes in young people's behavior. In contrast, evidence presented by supporters of comprehensive sexuality education focused exclusively on extensive quantitative research showing that comprehensive sexuality education reduces teen pregnancy and does not encourage earlier ages of sexual initiation. No testimonials were included. As a result of these Senate hearings, abstinence-only education remained the only federally-funded sexuality education at that time (Tolman et al. 2005).

Tolman et al. (2005) further articulated that the traditional conventions of rigor usually affect policy-makers through the use of scientific evidence and uphold that statistics are the only form of real data. However, the compelling voices of adolescents could provide countervailing persuasive stories to the debate or, quite possibly, change its terms altogether. Testimonials have become a powerful part of the political process, because stories are persuasive and can likely move politicians to make policies that reflect the experiences conveyed. The disadvantage is that testimonials do not represent the variety and complexity of any human experience (Tolman et al. 2005). Rather, the methodo-logically rigorous techniques of qualitative methods provide a way to study the depth of human thought, experience, and decision-making. Listening to stories or narratives from a variety of people, for example, may identify and illuminate social patterns and unique individual experiences that can help influence policy-makers' decisions. The researchers found from key findings of qualitative research studies that the sexuality education debate has left out central, developmental, and interpersonal aspects of girls' sexuality (Tolman et al. 2005).

10.2.4 Policy on Family Presence as a Recommendation from a Phenomenological Study in the ICU

The phenomenological research I conducted in 2010 explored the lived experiences of patients, their family members, and their nurses during critical illness in the ICU (Cypress 2010). It affirmed the mutual influence among family members, patient, and nurses during a critical illness experience and supported the tenets of family-centered care, which mandate the purposeful inclusion of the family in all aspects of care. As a result of this study, I drafted a policy on family presence during invasive and emergency procedures, which was submitted to the ICU in the institution where the inquiry was conducted and is reproduced here.

10.2.4.1 Family Presence Policy in the Intensive Care Unit

- Practice statement: Family members will be permitted in the patient care area during either invasive procedures or emergency situations like resuscitation.
- Purpose: To provide patients and families care that is consistent with the philosophy of family-centered care.

Definitions

- Invasive procedure: Any intervention that involves manipulation of the body or penetration of the body's natural barriers to the external environment (MacLean et al. 2003).
- Resuscitation: A sequence of events, including invasive and emergency procedures, which are initiated to sustain life or prevent further deterioration of the patient's condition.
- Family: A relative of the patient or any person (significant other) with whom the patient shares an established relationship (MacLean et al. 2003).
- Family presence: The attendance of family members in a location that affords visual or physical contact with the patient during invasive procedures or resuscitation.
- Family facilitator: A staff member (nurse, physician, chaplain, social worker, child life specialist, physician assistant, trained volunteers, and other health-care team member) assigned specifically to initiate interventions that assist the family and provide emotional and psychosocial support.

Procedures

1. The healthcare team will be responsible for assessing patient and family needs for visitation during invasive, emergency procedures, or resuscitation efforts in selected situations.

2. When family members are being given information about the patient's status, response to treatment, and identified needs, staff shall participate with the family facilitator in evaluating whether families are suitable candidates for bedside visitation. Before the family presence option is offered, families will be assessed for appropriate levels of coping and the absence of combative behavior, extreme emotional instability or outbursts, and behaviors consistent with altered mental status form effects of drugs, alcohol or those suspected of abuse.

3. If the direct care providers agree that family visitation is possible, the patient will be asked (if conscious) if he or she wishes to have a family member present. If the patient and direct care providers agree, then the family will be offered the option of family presence. When prioritizing family member's visitation and determining the next of kin, the consent for medical treatment guidelines will be used by the staff. Routinely two people (depending on assessment of individual needs) will be allowed in the room. Family members who do not wish to participate shall be supported in their decision.

4. Before entering the patient care area, the family facilitator will explain about the patient's appearance, treatments, and equipment used in the care room. The family facilitator will prepare the family for entering the patient care area by communicating that patient care is the priority, and then explaining how many family members may enter the room, where they may stand, situations in which they would be escorted out of the room (such as unexpected patient events or family becoming overwhelmed or disruptive), possible time restrictions, when they may leave the room, and any other pertinent factors.

5. The family member(s) will enter the patient care area escorted by the family facilitator. If appropriate, the family member(s) will be provided with personal protective equipment and instructed on its use. They will also be informed of where to stand and what not to touch to prevent contaminating the patient or supplies during a sterile procedure.

6. The family facilitator will:
   - explain interventions;
   - interpret medical or nursing jargon;
   - provide information about expected outcomes or the patient's response to treatment;
   - supply comfort measures, such as a chair at the patient's bedside or tissues;
   - give an opportunity to ask questions;
   - grant an opportunity to see, touch, and speak to the patient.

7. If a family member faints, becomes hysterical, or disruptive at the bedside, the family facilitator will immediately escort him or her from the area and arrange appropriate supportive care.

8. After completing the patient visit, the facilitator will escort the family to a comfortable area, address their concerns, provide comfort measures, and address other psychosocial needs identified during the intervention.
9. If staff involved in family presence identifies the need for debriefing regarding the case, the area supervisor will be informed to make a referral to the critical incident stress management team coordinator or patient relations officer.
10. The family facilitator will also communicate need for family follow-up to the bereavement care team.

10.3 Phenomenological Research and Knowledge and Theory Development

Research as a whole is a means by which discoveries are made, ideas are confirmed or refuted, and theories are developed and refined. All of these factors contribute to development of knowledge (Morse and Field 1995). Both quantitative and qualitative research are tools for solving research problems. Quantitative research studies phenomena that have been examined by researchers possessing prior knowledge from which to work and means of measuring variables and testing a theory. Qualitative research is the primary means by which the theoretical foundations of social science may be constructed and reexamined (Morse and Field 1995). It is usually conducted to explore problems about which little is known. Qualitative researchers primarily aim to develop or construct a description of an observed phenomenon in order to generate a solid theory as the outcome or product of the research. Instead of constructing theoretical framework from which to work deductively, they approach the inquiry inductively (Morse and Field, 1995, p. 4).

10.3.1 Function of Theory

A theory is a hunch, a guess, a speculation, or an idea that may explain a reality. It is also a systematic explanation of an event in which constructs and concepts are identified, relationships are proposed, and predictions are made (Morse and Field 1995; Strauss and Corbin 1994). The inductive approach of qualitative research allows the researcher to examine data for patterns and relationships and to develop hypotheses to generate a theory. Theory narrows and more fully specifies the phenomenon of interest and provides a relatively concrete and specific structure for the interpretation of initially puzzling behaviors, situations, and events (Fawcett 2000, p. 19). Furthermore, because theory is inductively derived, it is quite likely to be right, and it can direct inquiry within a particular discipline (Morse and Field 1995).

Morse and Field (1995) present seven functions of theory in knowledge development: (i) theory builds tension within a discipline as it initiates debate and dialogue; (ii) theory is a counter-nihilism as it fills gaps in knowledge and combats "intellectual nothingness"; (iii) theory is temporality as it places phenomena in time, anchoring observations in relation to nature and history; (iv) theory clarifies and provides explanations for otherwise seemingly unrelated facts; (v) theory predicts events and outcomes and guides investigations; (vi) theory reveals or discloses and draws attention to a particular phenomenon; and (vii) theory silences an area by ignoring phenomena. Thus, theory has an important role for science and society (Morse and Field 1995). A developed theory from qualitative research may serve important functions within a discipline as it provides insights that revise or alter clinical practice (Morse and Field 1995). What qualitative approaches can knowledge be derived from that will help with theory development? Synthesis of qualitative evidence is one of the ways in which new knowledge can be obtained.

10.3.2 Synthesis of Qualitative Research and Knowledge Development

The contribution of qualitative evidence to healthcare decision-making is increasingly acknowledged. Synthesis of qualitative research has been ongoing since the 1980s. The "urge to synthesize" can be situated within three important trends: the explosion of qualitative research studies, the rise of evidence-based practice, and the perceived underuse and undervaluation of the current body of qualitative research results (Sandelowski and Barroso 2007). A synthesis may offer valuable information such as contextually distinct findings that can be added to the evidence base and used by policy-makers and practitioners (Finfgeld-Connett 2010) to improve patient care (Finfgeld-Connett 2010). Qualitative evidence synthesis (**QES**) – the preferred umbrella term of the Cochrane Qualitative & Implementation Methods Group for over 20 different methods of qualitative synthesis – now occupies an important role within the activities of international collaborations such as the British National Institute for Health and Clinical Excellence (**NICE**) and the U.S. Agency for Healthcare Research and Quality (**AHRQ**). The Cochrane Collaboration's Qualitative & Implementation Methods Group was formally recognized in 2006, and the first Cochrane QES was published in 2013.

10.3.3 The Cochrane Qualitative & Implementation Methods Group

The Cochrane Qualitative & Implementation Methods Group focuses on methods and processes involved in the synthesis and integration of qualitative evidence. It aims to advise the Cochrane organization and its network on policy and practice, develop and maintain methodological guidance, and provide training to those undertaking Cochrane reviews (Cochrane Qualitative & Implementation Methods Group 2020).

There are four ways that qualitative research can potentially contribute to Cochrane Intervention reviews: (i) informing reviews by using evidence from qualitative research to help define and refine the research question, to ensure the review includes appropriate studies and addresses important outcomes; (ii) enhancing reviews by synthesizing evidence from qualitative research identified while looking for evidence of effectiveness; (iii) extending reviews by undertaking a search to specifically seek out evidence from qualitative studies to address questions directly related to the effectiveness review; and

(iv) supplementing reviews by synthesizing qualitative evidence within a standalone, but complementary, qualitative review to address questions on aspects other than effectiveness (Noyes and Lewin 2011).

Identifying and reviewing qualitative research can produce relevant information about populations, interventions, outcomes, and the relationship between these during the development of a protocol for a Cochrane systematic review of effectiveness. There are other advantages to the use of qualitative evidence in reviews, related to producing information that: (i) can help make decisions about the characteristics of people or a population; (ii) inform the development of robust effectiveness questions and protocols that may influence effectiveness; (iii) help with issues such as health perceptions, understanding of the intervention, preferences for treatment options, accessibility, and perceptions of acceptable/important outcomes that can be used to inform decisions about subgroup analysis as the protocol is being developed; and (iv) help to identify secondary review questions to be specified in the protocol (Harris 2011).

10.3.4 Approaches to Qualitative Evidence Synthesis

There have been an increasing number of QES papers appearing in the healthcare literature. QES methods have the potential to generate answers to complex questions that provide us with novel, valuable insights for theory development and clinical practice (Benoot et al. 2016). Milestones for the development of QES methodology are well documented, but not without challenges, debate, and discussion. This relates to the question of whether qualitative studies should be synthesized, and how; the confusing terminologies; the issue of rigor; and the various methods available to assess these naturalistic inquiries. Methodologists tend to define and organize synthesis approaches on a spectrum from integrative/aggregative/summative to interpretive and theory-generating (Noblit and Hare 1988; Noyes and Lewin 2011).

10.3.4.1 Integrative/Aggregative/Summative Synthesis

Integrative/aggregative/summative syntheses are "conventional" systematic reviews focused on amalgamating, combining, assembling, pooling, and summarizing data with the assumption that the concepts (or variables) under which those data are to be summarized are largely secure and well specified (Dixon-Woods et al. 2005; Noyes and Lewin 2011). The aim is to assess evidence and test hypotheses for causality (theory-testing). This requires a basic comparability between phenomena so that the data can be aggregated for analysis. Key concepts are defined at an early stage in the review and form the categories under which the data from empirical studies can be summarized (Noyes and Lewin 2011). If the goal is theory generation, however, then integration, aggregation, and summation are not the appropriate approaches; rather, interpretation (interpretive synthesis) and theory development should be used.

10.3.4.2 Interpretive and Theory-Generating Synthesis

Interpretive and theory-generating syntheses see the essential tasks of synthesis as involving both induction and interpretation toward the generation and evolution of the concepts of analysis into a higher-order theoretical structure and the development of theories that integrate those concepts (Dixon-Woods et al. 2005). The purpose is the generation of a synthesizing argument – a theory. Concepts are generally not specified in advance of the synthesis; rather, they emerge as a product of the interpretive analysis (Noyes and Lewin 2011). Sampling (theoretical) involves a highly iterative constant dialectic process concurrent with theory generation. The development of theoretical categories is based on an analysis of conceptual similarities and differences identified in the literature, and a constant comparison across them. The analysis that yields the synthesis is conceptual in process and output, and the product is not aggregations of data, but theory. A middle-range theory or explanation that applies in a specified domain can also be generated, which may address questions not answered through integrative synthesis (Dixon-Woods et al. 2005; Noyes and Lewin 2011). Some examples of primarily qualitative and interpretive approaches are metaethnography, critical interpretive synthesis, narrative summary, realist synthesis, metanarrative mapping, grounded theory, Miles and Huberman's techniques (Dixon-Woods et al. 2005), and qualitative metasynthesis. Metasynthesis may be a metaethnography (interpretive comparison of study findings) (Noblit and Hare 1988), a meta-study (critical/discursive engagement with data) (Paterson et al. 2001), or a qualitative research synthesis (**QRS**) (integrating research findings through a meta-summary or metasynthesis) (Sandelowski and Barroso 2007).

10.3.5 Metasynthesis and Theory Construction

Qualitative metasynthesis attempts to integrate results from multiple different but interrelated qualitative studies with interpretive, rather than aggregating, intent – in contrast to meta-analysis of quantitative studies (Walsh and Downe 2005). It is an interpretive integration of qualitative findings that are themselves interpretive syntheses of data, including phenomenology, ethnography, grounded theory, and other integrated and coherent descriptions or explanations of phenomena, events, or cases (Sandelowski and Barroso 2007). Metasynthesis is the bringing together and breaking down of findings, their examination, the discovery of essential features, and, in some way, the combining of phenomena into a transformed whole (Schreiber et al. 1997). Sandelowski et al. (2004) consider qualitative metasynthesis as one kind of systematic review and a type of qualitative research integration. Moreover, metasynthesis is not a method designed to produce oversimplification; rather, it is one with a goal that is clearly interpretive, in which differences are retained and complexity is enlightened (Thorne et al. 2004). The purpose of qualitative metasynthesis is theory building, theory development, and higher-level abstraction (Cypress and Frederickson 2017). Theory building is the bringing of findings to a theoretical level, or tentative theory. Qualitative metasynthesis also seeks to develop and refine theories (theory explication) while retaining the particularity of individual studies. Theory explication is the reconceptualization of the original phenomenon – a single concept. A sample metasynthesis as an outcome inspired by two phenomenological research studies previously conducted in the ICU and ED will be presented by way of demonstration.

10.3.6 Family Presence in the ICU and ED: A Metasynthesis

In 2017, I conducted a metasynthesis of findings from 17 qualitative research inquiries on family presence and the experiences of nurses, patients, and family members, guided by Sandelowski and Barroso's (2007) approach (Cypress and Frederickson 2017). The review of literature showed that there were a number of quantitative meta-analyses but no metasynthesis of qualitative studies on family presence in critical-care areas, or specifically in these two acute settings, during the 10-year period from 2004–2013. Further, most studies on family presence have primarily focused on presence during cardiopulmonary resuscitation (**CPR**).

Family presence for this metasynthesis is defined as the inclusion of family members during and following acute events such as CPR and invasive procedures, family conferences, rounds, nursing and patient care, withdrawal of life-sustaining therapy, and the process of dying in the ICU and ED. The essential themes of emotional support, feelings of safety and comfort, knowing, understanding, being informed, and being engaged emerged from the review synthesis. Being present with the patient and knowing the health condition, prognosis, and possible outcomes strengthen the whole family. It allows them to endure, adapt positively, and deal with suffering by sustaining energy and hope, finding meaning in the situation, striving for consolation, and trying to rebuild life under new conditions. An overarching theme of family coping during stressful times such as hospitalization is described as "system support," and is noted in the literature as a component of *family resilience*. Although there were no specific measures of the effect of supportive behaviors on family function in the studies included in this metasynthesis, when examined according to family resilience theory, elements necessary to resilience were present. The outcomes that emerged were reports by families of the general effects of support, such as "assisted with decision-making," "knowing what was going on as an active participant," "presence with CPR assisted grieving," and "served as an advocate when I couldn't think." In critical-care situations, positive relationships among family members, nurses, and patients allow for healing and growth among the triad, as nurses and direct-care providers promote family resilience – an opportunity rarely available to other healthcare providers but one that is important for the development of a theory of family resilience in critical-care settings (Cypress and Frederickson 2017).

This study adds to already compelling evidence in support of family presence in critical care. The findings also extend those of investigations supporting the inclusion of family presence in hospitals' formal written policies and protocols guiding provider practice in the ICU and ED. This metasynthesis provides an opportunity to test Masten and Coatsworth's (1998) three-part model of resilience by deriving a number of propositions. Future research on family presence in the ICU and ED is recommended to test these three propositions: (i) a health-related critical event, a time of significant risk, creates a unique opportunity for professionals to provide protective resources; (ii) family presence during life-altering treatments, regardless of the medical outcome, provides a calming effect through knowing changes in status; and (iii) providing specific protective support during a health-related critical event promotes family resilience. The researchers also recommend that further studies be conducted to relate supportive behaviors of critical care nurses to family functioning and provide empirical evidence for further development of the theory of family resilience (Cypress and Frederickson 2017).

10.4 Conclusion

This chapter discussed the utility of qualitative research findings and their linkage to outcomes specifically in EBP, policy, and theory. It presented the topics of asking "meaning questions" in evidence-based reviews, policy as an outcome of phenomenological research, and knowledge and theory development gained through this naturalistic research approach.

References

American College of Critical Care Medicine. (2017). Family-centered care in ICU. Available from https://www.sccm.org/Research/Guidelines/Guidelines/Family-Centered-Care-in-the-ICU (accessed May 10, 2021).

Benoot, C., Hansen, K., and Bilsen, J. (2016). The use of purposeful sampling in a qualitative evidence synthesis: a worked example on sexual adjustment to a cancer trajectory. BMC Medical Research Methodology 16 (21): 1–12.

Brantlinger, E., Jimenez, R., Klingner, J. et al. (2005). Qualitative studies in special education. Exceptional Children 71 (2): 95–207.

Brown, K.N., Leigh, J.P., Kamran, H. et al. (2018). Transfers from intensive care unit to hospital ward: a multicentre textual analysis of physician progress notes. Critical Care 22 (1): 19.

Buchner, D.L., Bagshaw, S.M., Dodek, P. et al. (2015). Prospective cohort study protocol to describe the transfer of patients from intensive care units to hospital wards. BMJ Open 5 (7): e007913.

Cochrane Qualitative & Implementation Methods Group. (2020). Homepage. Available from https://methods.cochrane.org/qi/welcome (accessed May 10, 2021).

Cooke, A., Smith, D., and Booth, A. (2012). Beyond PICO: the SPIDER tool for qualitative evidence synthesis. Qualitative Health Research 22 (10): 1435–1445.

Cypress, B. (2010). The intensive care unit: experiences of patients, families, and their nurses. Dimensions of Critical Care Nursing 29 (2): 94–101.

Cypress, B. (2011). Family conference in the intensive care unit: a systematic review. Dimensions of Critical Care Nursing 30 (5): 246–255.

Cypress, B. (2012). Family presence in rounds: an evidence-based review. Dimensions of Critical Care Nursing 31 (1): 53–63.

Cypress, B. (2013). Transfer out of intensive care: an evidence-based literature review. Dimensions of Critical Care Nursing 32 (5): 244–261.

Cypress, B. (2015). Qualitative research: the "what," "why," "who," and "how"! Dimensions of Critical Care Nursing 34 (6): 356–361.

Cypress, B. and Frederickson, K. (2017). Family presence in the intensive care unit and emergency department: a metasynthesis. Journal of Family Theory and Practice 9 (2): 201–218.

Daniels, K., Loewenson, R., George, A. et al. (2016). Fair publication of qualitative research in health systems: a call by health policy and systems researchers. International Journal for Equity in Health 15 (98): 1–9.

Davidson, J., Aslakson, R.A., Long, A.C. et al. (2017). Guidelines for family-centered care in the neonatal, pediatric, and adult ICU. Critical Care Medicine 45 (1): 104–128.

Dixon-Woods, M., Agarwal, S., Jones, D. et al. (2005). Synthesizing qualitative and quantitative evidence: a review of possible methods. Journal of Health Services Research Policy 10 (1): 45B–53B.

Dumas, M.J. and Anderson, G. (2014). Qualitative research as policy knowledge: framing policy problems and transforming education from the ground up. Education Policy Analysis Archives 22 (11): 10.14507.

Elliott, R.A., Lee, C.Y., Beanland, C. et al. (2017). Development of a clinical pharmacy model within an Australian home nursing service using co-creation and participatory action research: the Visiting Pharmacist (ViP) study. BMJ Open 7: e018722. 1–10.

Estabrooks, C.A. (1999a). The conceptual structure of research utilization. Research in Nursing and Health 22 (2): 203–216.

Estabrooks, C.A. (1999b). Will evidence-based nursing practice make practice perfect? Canadian Journal of Nursing Research 30 (1): 273–294.

Fawcett, J. (2000). Analysis and Evaluation of Contemporary Nursing Knowledge: Nursing Models and Theories. F. A. Davis Company.

Finfgeld-Connett, D. (2010). Generalizability and transferability of meta-synthesis research findings. Journal of Advanced Nursing 6 (2): 246–254.

Gopalakrishnan, S. and Ganeshkumar, P. (2013). Systematic reviews and meta-analysis: understanding the best evidence in primary healthcare. Journal of Family Medicine and Primary Care 2 (1): 9–14.

Graham, H. and McDermott, E. (2016). Qualitative research and the evidence base of policy: insights from studies of teenage mothers in the UK. Journal of Social Policy 35 (1): 21–37.

Harris, J. (2011). Using qualitative research to develop robust effectiveness questions and protocols for Cochrane systematic reviews. In: Supplementary Guidance for Inclusion of Qualitative Research in Cochrane Systematic Reviews of Interventions, version 1 (updated August 2011) (eds. J. Noyes, A. Booth, K. Hannes, et al.). Cochrane Collaboration Qualitative Methods Group.

Hurd, C.J. and Curtis, J.R. (2015). The intensive care unit family conference teaching a critical intensive care unit procedure. Annals of American Thoracic Society 12 (4): 469–471.

Institute of Medicine. (2011). Finding what works in health care: standards for systematic reviews. Available from http://www.nap.edu/catalog/13059/finding-what-works-in-health-care-standards-for-systematic-reviews (accessed May 10, 2021).

Jack, S. (2006). Utility of qualitative research findings in evidence-based public health practice. Public Health Nursing 23 (3): 277–283.

Jodaki, K., Ghyasvandian, S., Abbasi, M. et al. (2017). Effect of Liaison nurse service on transfer anxiety of patients transferred from the cardiac surgery intensive care unit to the general ward. Nursing and Midwifery Studies 6 (1): e33478. 1–4.

Kearney, M.H. (1998). Ready to wear: discovering grounded formal theory. Research in Nursing & Health 21: 179–186.

Kearney, M.H. (2001). Focus on research methods: levels and applications of qualitative research evidence. Research in Nursing and Health 24: 145–153.

Kodali, S. (2014). Family experience with intensive care unit care: association of self-reported family conferences and family satisfaction. Journal of Critical Care 29 (4): 641–644.

Kozleski, E. (2017). The uses of qualitative research: powerful methods to inform evidence-based practice in education. Research and Practice Persons with Severe Disabilities 42 (1): 19–32.

Kramer, A.A., Higgins, T.L., and Zimmerman, J.E. (2013). The association between ICU readmission rate and patient outcomes. Critical Care Medicine 41 (1): 24–33.

MacLean, S.L., Guzzetta, C.E., White, C. et al. (2003). Family presence during cardiopulmonary resuscitation and invasive procedures: practices of critical care and emergency nurses. Journal of Emergency Nursing 29 (3): 208–221.

Masten, A.S. and Coatsworth, J.D. (1998). The development of competence in favorable and unfavorable environments: lessons from research on successful children. American Psychologist 53 (2): 205–220.

Melnyk, B.M. and Fineout-Overholt, E. (2019). Evidence-Based Practice in Nursing and Healthcare, 4e. Lippincott Williams & Wilkins.

Miller, W. (2010). Qualitative research findings as evidence: utility in nursing practice. Clinical Nurse Specialist 24 (4): 91–193.

Morris, S., Wooding, S., and Grant, J. (2011). The answer is 17 years, what is the question: understanding time lags in translational research. Journal of the Royal Society of Medicine 104 (12): 510–520.

Morse, J. (1997). Completing a Qualitative Project: Details and Dialogue. Sage Publications.

Morse, J.M. (2001). Qualitative verification: building evidence by extending basic findings. In: The Nature of Qualitative Evidence (eds. J.M. Morse, J.M. Swanson and A.J. Kuzel), 203–220. Sage Publications.

Morse, J. and Field, P.A. (1995). Qualitative Research Methods for Health Professionals, 2e. Sage Publications.

Morse, J.M., Hutchinson, S.A., and Penrod, J. (1998). From theory to practice: the development of assessment guides from qualitatively derived theory. Qualitative Health Research 8 (3): 329–340.

Muecke, M.A. (1997). Policy as forethought in qualitative research: a paradigm from developing country social scientists. In: Completing a Qualitative Project: Details and Dialogue (ed. J. Morse), 357–379. Sage Publications.

National Transitions of Care Coalition. (2020). Improving transitions of care. Available from http://www.ntocc.org/Portals/0/PDF/Resources/PolicyPaper.pdf (accessed May 10, 2021).

Noblit, G. and Hare, R. (1988). Meta-Ethnography: Synthesizing Qualitative Studies. Sage Publications.

Nordgren, L., Asp, M., and Fagerberg, I. (2008). The use of qualitative evidence in clinical care. Evidence-Based Nursing 11 (1): 4–5.

Noyes, J. (2010). Never mind the qualitative feel the depth! The evolving role of qualitative research in Cochrane intervention reviews. Journal of Research in Nursing 15 (6): 525–534.

Noyes, J. and Lewin, S. (2011). Supplemental guidance on selecting a method of qualitative evidence synthesis, and integrating qualitative evidence with cochrane intervention reviews. In: Supplementary Guidance for Inclusion of Qualitative Research in Cochrane Systematic Reviews of Interventions, version 1 (updated August 2011) (eds. J. Noyes, A. Booth, K. Hannes, et al.). Cochrane Collaboration Qualitative Methods Group.

Odom, S.L. (2009). The tie that binds: evidence-based practice, implementation science, and outcomes for children. Topics Early Childhood Special Education 29 (1): 53–61.

Olson, K. (2001). Using qualitative research in clinical practice. In: The Nature of Qualitative Evidence (eds. J.M. Morse, J.M. Swanson and A.J. Kuzel), 259–273. Sage Publications.

Paterson, B.L., Thorne, S., Canam, C., and Jillings, C. (2001). Meta-Study of Qualitative Health Research: A Practical Guide to Meta-Analysis and Metasynthesis. Sage Publications.

Pearson, A. (2010). Evidence-based healthcare and qualitative research. Journal of Research in Nursing 15 (6): 489–493.

Roberts, A.E. and Barber, G. (2001). Applying research evidence to practice. British Journal of Occupational Therapy 64 (5): 223–227.

Sandelowski, M. (2004). Using qualitative research. Qualitative Health Research 14 (10): 1366–1386.

Sandelowski, M. and Barroso, J. (2003). Classifying the findings in qualitative studies. Qualitative Health Research 13 (7): 905–923.

Sandelowski, M. and Barroso, J. (2007). Handbook for Synthesizing Qualitative Research. Springer.

Sandelowski, M. and Leeman, L. (2012). Practice-based evidence and qualitative inquiry. Journal of Nursing Scholarship 44 (2): 171–179.

Schreiber, R., Crooks, D., and Stern, P.N. (1997). Qualitative meta-analysis. In: Completing a Qualitative Project: Details and Dialogue (ed. J.M. Morse), 311–326. Sage Publications.

Scottish Intercollegiate Guidelines Network (2008). SIGN 50. A Guidelines Developers Handbook. SIGN Executive.

Squires, A. and Dorsen, C. (2018). Qualitative research in nursing and health professions regulation. Journal of Nursing Regulation 9 (3): 15–24.

Stelfox, H.T., Leigh, J.P., Dodek, P.M. et al. (2017). A multi-center prospective cohort study of patient transfers from the intensive care unit to the hospital ward. Intensive Care Medicine 43 (10): 1485–1494.

Strauss, A. and Corbin, J. (1994). Grounded theory methodology: an overview. In: Hand Book of Qualitative Research (eds. N. Denzin and Y. Lincoln), 262–272. Sage.

Thorne, S.E. (2001). The implications of disciplinary agenda on quality criteria for qualitative research. In: The Nature of Qualitative Evidence (eds. J.M. Morse, J. Swanson and A. Kuzel), 141–159. Sage Publications.

Thorne, S., Jensen, L., Kearney, M.H. et al. (2004). Qualitative metasynthesis: reflections on methodological orientation and ideological agenda. Qualitative Health Research 14 (10): 1342–1365.

Tolman, D., Hirschman, C., and Impett, E.A. (2005). There is more to the story: the place of qualitative research on female adolescent sexuality in policy making. Sexuality Research and Social Policy: Journal of NSRC 2 (4): 4–17.

Walsh, D. and Downe, S. (2005). Meta-synthesis method for qualitative research: a literature review. Journal of Advanced Nursing 50 (2): 204–211.

Index

Page locators in **bold** indicate tables. Page locators in *italics* indicate figures. This index uses letter-by-letter alphabetization.